Dear Ellen

One of my most
successful clients!

Urban Skinny

Thank you for
your support!

♡ Danïelle Schupp

Urban Skinny

Live the Fabulous Life–
and Still Zip Up Your
Favorite Jeans

Danielle Schupp, RD, with Stephanie Krikorian

Guilford, Connecticut

GPP Life is an imprint of The Globe Pequot Press.

Urban Skinny is a registered trademark of Danielle Schupp and Stephanie Krikorian.

Text design: Libby Kingsbury
Project manager: Lara Asher

Library of Congress Cataloging-in-Publication Data

Schupp, Danielle.
  Urban skinny : live the fabulous life—and still zip up your favorite jeans / Danielle Schupp ; with Stephanie Krikorian.
     p. cm.
  ISBN 978-0-7627-5079-5
  1. Weight loss. 2. Urban women—Health and hygiene. I. Krikorian, Stephanie. II. Title.
  RM222.2.S352 2010
  613.2'5—dc22
                                                                                    2009018289

Printed in the United States of America

10 9 8 7 6 5 4 3 2 1

Contents

To never having to say "I'll start Monday" again

Diet Is a
Four-Letter Word,
Even in New York City

The Urban Skinny plan is not a diet. (Yeah, yeah—you've heard that before.) Urban Skinny will teach you how to work any city, not have the city work you over. It will take you from just plain urban to fabulously Urban Skinny. It won't tell you how to *avoid* urban culinary temptations; it will show you how to navigate them and indulge in all a city has to offer while still being able to zip up those True Religions. Urban Skinny is all about strategy—it's a livable plan for city dwellers with busy work and social lives. It isn't about being perfect—it's about being consistent with your eating and working through every challenging situation you may encounter when you live a jam-packed urban lifestyle.

My name is Danielle Schupp and I'm a registered dietitian at one of the hottest health clubs in Manhattan—Reebok Sports Club/NY. I counsel fifty to sixty clients a week, helping them manage their weight and feel great about how they look and feel. Some people come to see me on their doctor's orders; some just want to squeeze into a smaller size. Many of my clients, especially the actors and pro athletes, want not only to look great, but also to keep up their energy during grueling fourteen-hour shoots and hard-core workout schedules. My clients come from all corners of the country and the world, and all over New York—SoHo, the Village, the Upper East and Upper West Sides. They're Wall Street power brokers, lawyers, doctors, writers, TV producers, actors, international financiers, models, and those on their way to the top. Their lives vary, but they all share some common threads. They're extremely smart, successful, driven, hard-working, health-conscious, social, part-of-the-scene, hip city dwellers. They work insane hours, they hold demanding, high-stress positions, and they want the best of the best—and they want it now. They rarely cook because they're too busy and they have the best restaurants in the world at their fingertips, and they embrace the food, culture, and pace that the big city has to offer. They eat out for fun and work, they attend the theater, and they hit major galas, movie premieres, and gallery openings. They've walked the red carpet or come damn close.

Before Urban Skinny they shared one gigantic problem: They tried every single fad diet in existence and they failed every single time. My clients are able to run hedge funds worth billions, produce Emmy-winning TV shows, and represent major corporate clients, but before they met me, they couldn't seem to lose weight. They couldn't get rid of that irritating last ten pounds or that full-fledged fifty. And though every once in a while they may have lightened their load, the pounds never stayed off. For such driven people, it was incredibly frustrating that they couldn't make it happen on their own. They did not understand why their work ethic—work hard, accomplish your goals—didn't necessarily apply to losing weight. Recognize yourself? Are you one of these people who can accomplish goals professionally and personally but can't lose weight?

Up until now, you were probably trying to alter your life to fit into your diet. No need. You probably know the science of weight loss by now—calories in versus calories out. Now you just need to change your plan, accept your lifestyle, and work on consistency and the Urban Skinny strategy. Believe it: You can seamlessly lose weight and stay on the move. You don't need to beat yourself up anymore for being unable to accomplish your weight-loss goals.

Over the years, I've invested a lot of time in gaining an understanding of what goes on in the corporate world, the legal one, and that of many other high-stress, high-stakes professions. Knowing what my clients are up against at work every day has helped me understand their food challenges—when they're meeting, how long their days end up stretching, where they eat, and what social demands they face—all factors that have added to their weight-loss struggles. I've sorted through hundreds of menus from high-end restaurants around the world, helping them figure out what to order and how to eat on the run. If they don't cook, I don't teach them to cook—I teach them to eat out strategically. I text them, phone them, and coach them to help make weight management a lifetime achievement, not just a short-term goal.

After years of being egged on by clients to put something in writing, I finally got it together. I've teamed up with one of my clients, writer and television producer Stephanie Krikorian, to turn my daily work into a fun, easy-to-follow book. Stephanie's battled her weight since she moved to New York City. Like so many new to the city, she gained pounds when she discovered there were so many great places to eat. She traveled regularly for work and got overwhelmed with juggling her diet with her love of food. Writing *Urban Skinny* with Stephanie was insightful—for both of us. As we sketched out the book we spent a lot of time discussing the "dieter" mentality. We had a good laugh going to restaurants around town looking at ordering from two different perspectives—that of a dieter and that of a dietitian. Stephanie's wit, combined with her understanding of how hard it is to keep her weight in check, along with my fifteen years of experience, makes *Urban Skinny* the real deal. Every chapter in the book starts with an example—a story of a successful client just like Stephanie and the battles he or she faced. I've used the anecdotal evidence of all of my clients and my knowledge of proven scientific evidence behind weight management to make these chapters comprehensive and informative. We've changed the names of everyone we write about, but their stories are all true. You can be one of these success stories, too.

Urban Skinny will dispel the Urban Myths and empower you to lose weight and keep it off—forever. Make today the last day you say

"I'll start Monday." There are no more Mondays. You're not going on a diet—you're changing the way you eat, but *not* changing the way you live. So if you can't make an appointment to see me, you can get the same insight and guidance by reading this book. Every word I've ever said to my clients over the years is in here somewhere.

> **Urban Skinny:** *In order to move forward and reach your weight goals, and more important, maintain a healthy weight, the first step is to stay positive. Most people think they suck at dieting. They don't realize that it's the diet they chose that sucked. People hope diets will give them a quick fix to a long-term problem. Weight management requires a lifelong commitment.* **Urban Skinny** *offers the solution with a long-range plan that doesn't slow down your life. It works food into your hectic schedule and fabulous lifestyle.*

So don't stay home in your pj's and drink lemon juice and maple syrup for ten days. Retreat is not the way to succeed at weight management. Go ahead and keep the reservation at the hottest spot in town. Just make sure you read *Urban Skinny* before you go out so you'll know how to indulge but not bulge! You can live large, but eat small.

Urban Skinny Rules—
Learn 'em, Live 'em!

- Breakfast is nonnegotiable. Eat it every day—no excuses.
- Order salad dressing on the side forevermore. Always.
- Smaller portions make smaller people.
- Enjoy dips, hummus, or fondue—but dip, don't dunk.
- Sip, don't slug, your alcohol.
- Don't drink your calories—wouldn't you rather eat an apple than drink juice?
- If you have wine with dinner, skip the bread, rice, or other starch.
- Get friendly with nonstick spray if you happen to catch yourself cooking at home—always use it.
- Be consistent, not perfect.
- Get your butt off the couch and exercise.

CHAPTER 1

There's No
Overdraft Protection
on Eating

Joanne, 28 years old, reality TV producer, started Urban Skinny at 200 pounds, lost 60 pounds, and has kept it off for three years.

Urban Challenge
Joanne works as a freelancer in a competitive TV business. Her hours are inconsistent—and so is what she puts in her mouth. When she's not working, things are okay, but when she gets a two-month TV gig, her eating goes haywire. She works twenty hours a day. She eats all her meals at work and throws food into her mouth whenever it's within sight. She eats late because she works late, and she skips breakfast because she's still full from eating dinner at 11:00 p.m. the night before. When it comes to food, she doesn't discriminate: If it gets delivered to the edit room, she eats it. Joanne uses food to cope with her high-pressure career, and she has no idea how many calories she's consuming.

Urban Surprise
Joanne still finds time to work out hard five times a week—with a trainer, no less!

Urban Insight
Joanne kept working out but figured out how many calories she should be consuming and started to plan and prepare meals to keep herself on track no matter how crazy her schedule got. She began eating breakfast and was able to cut her intake throughout the day as a result. Joanne scoped out restaurants and takeout places within a couple of blocks of work. She avoided group ordering and made her own delivery choices, which included salads and simple sandwiches. She pre-packed lunch on Mondays from her leftover Saturday takeout order and made sure she had a 200-calorie mid-afternoon healthy snack on hand every day. She used a lot of pre-measured frozen meals to keep herself honest. Joanne never winged it. She's not a winger. She needed the structure to keep herself in check.

Urban Skinny
Non–breakfast eaters overeat at night. Breakfast eaters are thinner.

Budget Your Calories

Forget carbs, forget fat. When you want to drop some pounds, the main thing you want to do is count your calories, and that's the bottom line. Like any financial budget, there's a weight-loss bottom line too, and it comes in the form of counted calories. The science is simple: calories in versus calories out. This chapter will help you figure out what you eat and how many calories you get to "spend" each day. Like a debit card with a spending limit, you get a certain amount of food each day. No more, no less.

URBAN INSIGHT: If you plan to drink, you don't get to eat as much. We know you're going to hit the town every once in a while. But remember that the more you drink, the less you should eat. (We do not, however, encourage you to drink heavily—especially on an empty stomach!) You might even find that since you have only so many calories to spend, you wind up forgoing the booze for food.

"Seriously, you're going to make me count calories?" That's what you're asking yourself right now, isn't it? You're saying, "Haven't hundreds of books already been written that claim to provide an easier way?" So many books have foods to phase out, foods to phase back in, and foods you can't even look at, never mind eat. Forget your preconceived notions, forbidden eats, and all the crazy point systems you've had to learn with other diets. Living within too many limits isn't going to help you manage your weight. Avoiding certain food groups won't help you long-term. Short-term, maybe you'll drop. But can you *live* a fabulous life if all you eat is dry tuna and mustard for lunch, or celery and lettuce one week then sweet potatoes the next? Honestly, are you going to live your life without a little aged Gouda and some vino? We think not. Calorie science is the framework, and it's the only proven way to lose weight and keep it off. But there's a strategy you need to engage in order to win. *Urban Skinny* is the playbook. In fact, it's the only game in town.

URBAN INSIGHT: Every day doesn't have to be a weight-loss day. If you finally get into Rao's, or you're celebrating your friend's divorce, eat. It's only one meal. But stop there. Once in a while you have to indulge, but it can't happen too often.

The first step to success is to figure out how many calories you're allowed each day. It's important to know how many calories you need, because if you eat too many you'll gain weight or never lose. Eating too few can be equally harmful. If you eat less than you should, over time you'll slow your metabolism (the rate at which your body burns calories), making weight loss even more challenging. Our bodies don't like to lose weight. If you under-eat, your body will learn to make do by becoming more efficient. That's the opposite of what you want to happen when you're trying to lose weight and maintain it. It also sets you up to feel deprived and can lead to binge eating, which causes the one thing you don't want to happen—weight gain. Initially, a big calorie reduction will cause rapid weight loss. But long-term, it will be harder and harder to reach your goal, and the likelihood of gaining the weight back increases because your metabolism slows down. The recommended weekly weight loss is one half to two pounds. Losing it any faster will make it harder to keep off and you will lose water and muscle, not just fat.

URBAN INSIGHT: When you cross the street, you look both ways. When you wake up in the morning, you brush your teeth. New life habit: When you order a salad, you get the dressing on the side. But hey, don't just pick it up and dump the whole thing on your salad—you ordered it on the side for a reason! Dip your fork in the dressing, then stab the lettuce.

Don't be afraid—counting calories isn't tedious. Just keep thinking about budgeting. You're a savvy professional; you budget your money. But maybe you use your credit card to buy a $500 outfit because the guy in the next office asked you out or you use overdraft protection to buy tickets to see Madonna in concert. If you're not a great budgeter, sometimes you spend more than you make, and you pay it back later. But there's no credit line with calories. Everything from the cream in your coffee to the dressing on your salad has calories that you're spending here and now, and there's no making up for it later. Special occasions are the one time you can calorie splurge, but most of the time you have to budget. Keeping track of your calories is easy, though—you just write everything down and do some simple math.

Urban Myth: *Counting calories is tedious and depressing, and it means being deprived.*

Urban Skinny: *The more you know and learn about calories, the more you can work your favorite foods into your healthy eating plan. Did you know ten tortilla chips and ½ cup of salsa have only 150 calories and provide you with a full serving of vegetables?*

Get Started with a Food Log

Keep a food log for a few days to a week just to see what you're eating. Keep a list of everything that goes in your mouth. You might be surprised at how much you're shoveling in. Don't alter your eating; just keep a running log so you'll be aware of how much your eating changes once you start Urban Skinny. Keep a running log throughout the day for accuracy; if you wait to write it all down at the end of the day, you'll forget too many things. You have to total your calories for each day. To get an idea of what you've eaten in calories, check the calorie lists we've included, read labels, and go to UrbanSkinny.com and other Web sites—Starbucks, Pinkberry, Subway, and most other chain restaurants post online the calorie counts for everything on their menus.

What you think you're eating and what you're actually eating aren't always in sync. You might not be an educated eater yet. But don't worry—by the time you've finished this book, you will be.

URBAN INSIGHT: Your food log will help you find out why you got where you are and what you need to do about it.

When you're reading a label, always check how large a serving is in addition to how many calories it has. For example, you may think a small bag of chips has only 150 calories, but that may be for only one serving when the bag actually holds two or three.

Nutrition Facts
(for a can of tuna)

Nutrition Facts

Serving Size 2 oz drained
(about ¼ cup)

Servings about 2.5

Calories 70	Fat Cal 10
Total Fat 1.0 g	2%
Cholesterol 25 mg	8%
Sodium 250mg	10%
Total Carb 0g	0%
Protein 15g	27%

Sample Food Log

Date: Wed., Jan. 28

Time	Food	Amount	Calories	Comment/ feelings
Breakfast 8:00 a.m.	Kashi cereal skim milk almonds berries	1 cup ½ cup 10 ½ cup	150 40 70 50//310	woke up hungry
Snack 10:15 a.m.	peach	small	60	feeling tired— needed snack
Lunch 12:00 p.m.	veg salad/ vinaigrette corn tuna nuts	1 ounce ½ cup 3 ounces 5	100 100 100 100 50//450	
Snack 4:00 p.m.	M&M's	bag	220	craving/late dinner planned
Subtotal			1,040	
Dinner 7:00 p.m.	chicken rice sauce on chicken	6 ounces ½ cup	200 100 100	felt full-tired/ craved sweet
Snack 9:00 p.m.	fruit cup	big looking	120	
Total Calories			1560	

H_2O—4 16-ounce bottles   Exercise—Yoga 90 min.

Go to UrbanSkinny.com to print this log, or use your own notebook to keep count, whichever works for you.

FOOD DIARY   **Date:**

Time	Food	Amount	Calories	Comment/ feelings
Subtotal				
Total Calories				

Now, after a few days of logging, take a look at how many calories you're eating and how many you *should be* eating. Find your range on the calorie chart on the next page—for example, if you are a 5'5" 30-year-old woman who is moderately active, aim to eat between 1500 and 1600 calories a day.

Write down how many calories you're allowed according to the chart. _____

You need to hit this number every day. You may need to tweak it ever so slightly, but we'll deal with that later when you reassess. So stick to it—it's an important number to get right. Having said that, plus or minus 50 calories a day is hitting your number. Don't get crazy over 25 or 30 calories.

Now start keeping that food log, but this time make sure each day you don't exceed your calorie number.

Write down everything as it's eaten. Track your food intake and the time and amount you eat, and record the calories of each item. You can print out a sample food log at UrbanSkinny.com. Don't write down everything at the end of the day. You might think you can remember it all, but you can't. You'll forget something and it will mess you up. When you eat it, note it, including beverages.

This may sound complicated, but it's truly easy—once you know the formula. As we've said, there's no overdraft protection when it comes to eating. You can average your calories out for the week, but you won't lose weight if you blow your calorie budget half the week.

As you read on, you'll realize this calorie allowance number might need to be tweaked slightly as your activity levels change or if you find yourself losing too quickly or too slowly. We'll teach you how to reassess later, but for now, get started with the number of calories you think best fits your profile.

Daily Caloric Chart

Note: If you are more than 100 pounds overweight, consult your doctor before starting any program.
*Minimum daily calorie intake for women is 1200.

WOMEN

		Sedentary	Moderately Active	Active	Very Active
Height 5'0"–5'1"	Age 20–40 | above 160 lbs. add 100 calories	1200–1300	1400–1500	1600–1700	1800–1900
	Age 40–60 |	*1200	1300–1400	1500–1600	1700–1800
Height 5'2"–5'3"	Age 20–40 | above 170 lbs. add 100 calories	1300–1400	1500–1600	1700–1800	1900–2000
	Age 40–60 |	1200–1300	1400–1500	1600–1700	1800–1900
Height 5'4"–5'5"	Age 20–40 | above 180 lbs. add 100 calories	1300–1400	1500–1600	1700–1800	1900–2000
	Age 40–60 |	1200–1300	1400–1500	1600–1700	1800–1900
Height 5'6"–5'7"	Age 20–40 | above 190 lbs. add 100 calories	1400–1500	1600–1700	1800–1900	2000–2100
	Age 40–60 |	1400–1500	1500–1600	1700–1800	1900–2000
Height 5'8"–5'9"	Age 20–40 | above 200 lbs. add 100 calories	1500–1600	1700–1800	1900–2000	2100–2200
	Age 40–60 |	1400–1500	1600–1700	1800–1900	2000–2100
Height 5'10"–5'11"	Age 20–40 | above 215 lbs. add 100 calories	1600–1700	1800–1900	2000–2100	2200–2300
	Age 40–60 |	1500–1600	1700–1800	1900–2000	2100–2200

Sedentary: no specific exercise program, < 1 mile walking throughout the day, office job

Moderately Active: exercise program 3 times per week, office job;
or no specific exercise routine but walks 2–3 miles per day every day

Active: exercises regularly 5–6 times per week, office job; or no specific exercise routine,
walks 4+ miles per day @ 15 minutes per mile, 5–6 times per week

Very Active: exercises 6 days per week @ high intensity for 60+ minutes; or exercises
more than once per day, e.g., triathletes, endurance athletes

Daily Caloric Chart

Note: If you are 100 pounds overweight, consult your doctor before starting any program.
*Minimum daily calorie intake for men is 1500.

MEN		Sedentary	Moderately Active	Active	Very Active
Height 5'4"–5'5"	Age 20–40 │ above 185 lbs. add 100 calories	1500–1600	1600–1900	2000–2100	2200–2300
	Age 40–60 │	*1500–1600	1700–1800	1900–2000	2100–2200
Height 5'6"–5'7"	Age 20–40 │ above 195 lbs. add 100 calories	1600–1700	1900–2000	2100–2200	2300–2400
	Age 40–60 │	1500–1600	1800–1900	2000–2100	2200–2300
Height 5'8"–5'9"	Age 20–40 │ above 210 lbs. add 100 calories	1700–1800	2000–2100	2200–2300	2400–2500
	Age 40–60 │	1600–1700	1900–2000	2100–2200	2300–2400
Height 5'10"–5'11"	Age 20–40 │ above 220 lbs. add 100 calories	1800–1900	2100–2200	2300–2400	2500–2600
	Age 40–60 │	1700–1800	2000–2100	2200–2300	2400–2500
Height 6'0"–6'1"	Age 20–40 │ above 235 lbs. add 100 calories	1900–2000	2200–2300	2400–2500	2600–2700
	Age 40–60 │	1800–1900	2100–2200	2300–1400	2500–2600
Height 6'2"–6'3"	Age 20–40 │ above 250 lbs. add 100 calories	2000–2100	2300–2400	2500–2600	2700–2800
	Age 40–60 │	1900–2000	2200–2300	2400–2500	2600–2700

Sedentary: no specific exercise program, < 1 mile walking throughout the day, office job

Moderately Active: exercise program 3 times per week, office job;
or no specific exercise routine but walks 2–3 miles per day every day

Active: exercises regularly 5–6 times per week, office job; or no specific exercise routine,
walks 4+ miles per day @ 15 minutes per mile, 5–6 times per week

Very Active: exercises 6 days per week @ high intensity for 60+ minutes; or exercises
more than once per day, e.g., triathletes, endurance athletes

Get Moving

This book is about eating and getting lean, but exercising is all a part of your success, so do some! Remember, calories in versus calories out. Here are a few great ways to burn some calories:

☐ Walk, run, bike, or swim

☐ Try yoga or pilates

☐ If you can afford it, hire a trainer

☐ If you don't like a traditional workout, try something like pole dancing at SFactor.com or take up tennis or surfing.

URBAN INSIGHT: **When 65-75% of your day is over, 65-75% of your eating should be over as well.**

Urban Myth: *Losing it fast is good.*

Urban Skinny: *The faster you lose it, the faster you gain it back. While it's true fast-paced New Yorkers want everything now, weight loss is the one thing in the Big Apple that does not happen in a New York minute.*

Urban Myth: *You can eat all your calories in one meal.*

Urban Skinny: *Spacing out your calories between small meals every three or four hours throughout the day helps rev up your metabolism.*

Organizing Your Food Allowance

Some diets let you hoard food until the end of the day. Not Urban Skinny. Don't starve all day so you can have a large order of pad thai, spring rolls, and two cocktails at dinner. You should spread out your calorie spending throughout the day to maximize your weight loss. Look at each meal listed below to find out what percentage of your total daily calories it should comprise.

> Urban Skinny Reminder
> Include protein and fat in every meal to stay full longer. It'll make those 1500 calories a *satisfying* 1500 calories rather than a *starving* 1500.

> ☐ *Breakfast:* 25% of total daily calories (within two hours of getting up). If you are working out before breakfast, eat a small piece of fruit first, and eat your breakfast when you're finished with the gym.
>
> ☐ *Lunch:* 25–30% of total daily calories
>
> ☐ *Snack:* 10–15% of total daily calories
>
> ☐ *Dinner:* 35% of total daily calories

So, for example, if your budget is 1500 calories in a day, eat 350–400 calories at breakfast, 400–500 calories at lunch, 100–200 calories for your snack, and 500–600 calories at dinner.

Urban Recap

Count calories, space your meals, include protein and fat in each meal, and keep a food log.

Up Next

Now that you know your calorie allowance, it's time to spend. What's more fun than spending—whether it's money or calories? That's the

Don't obsess about one goal weight. Weigh in—jump on the scale because you need a starting weight. Think in baby steps right now—one pound at a time. We'll discuss your "goal" later. And remember, the scale isn't your only measure of success—there are other ways we'll review later in the book.

next step in the Urban Skinny plan—knowing what you're eating, how you're spending what you have to spend, and how to make every calorie a worthwhile purchase. As you learn in the next chapter what you're spending, don't forget your water intake—try to get eight-plus glasses a day (or four sixteen-ounce bottles)! It's calorie free, so drink up. A gross little tip: If your pee is dark yellow, drink more water. Colorless or pale yellow is a sign of hydration.

CHAPTER 2

You Can't
Have Your Cosmo
and Eat
Your Cake, Too

Stephanie, writer, was on a weight-loss roller coaster, losing a lot of pounds over the years in 15- to 30-pound spurts. She always gained it back and then some until she started Urban Skinny. She now maintains within a 5-pound range of her goal weight.

Urban Challenge
Stephanie is a jet-setter. She'll go to Paris for a weekend and to the Cayman Islands for a week with two days' notice. She loves restaurants, and like any other single person, she either eats at home alone or she goes out to eat with friends. And the wine—she doesn't order by the glass but by the bottle. She takes comfort in a plate of truffle french fries the way some people might embrace their flannel pajamas. She likes going to the gym, and she loves to power walk, but she has no regular schedule and never fails to cancel her pretend workout plans for an invite to do, well, anything else. She may diet in spurts, but in general she never really pays much attention to how much she consumes and she's never consistent.

Urban Surprise
Stephanie rarely eats sweets. She never orders dessert, she can count on one hand the number of times she's bought ice cream, and if you

tore apart her apartment you still wouldn't find any hidden cookies or chocolate.

Urban Insight

Once Stephanie started a food log, she began learning just how much everything she ate was costing her in weight gain. She started skipping the crap the airlines handed her when she flew and instead packed her own bars and fruit. She passed on the bread basket because she certainly wasn't giving up the Bordeaux, and she ate breakfast at home — a perfect 350-calorie meal each morning. She hit the streets, making sure she walked sixty minutes a day, and added yoga to her workout regimen. She never ordered a pizza for delivery because she knew she would eat the entire thing, but she made sure she ate a slice once a week for lunch because it made her happy, tasted good, and curbed cravings.

Urban Skinny: *Depriving yourself of things you like only works short-term. Sooner or later, you'll fall and you'll fall hard. Enjoy a taste of your fave. Just measure it; don't eliminate it.*

Your Food Budget

So, you want to look great and be fabulous? You want to rock the social scene and still zip up your skinny jeans? Sounds like a challenge, but really it's not. You simply need to budget your food like you budget your money. Spend your food calories, but not like you spend your bonus. You can live the big-city life, hit the hot spots, eat power lunches, and make deals over drinks. You just need to be as savvy about what you're putting in your mouth as you are about your career.

If you want to lose weight, you can still go to your favorite restaurants and be social, but you need to know that if you insist on having two glasses of wine, you'll have to forfeit the fondue. If you just downed

300 calories in booze (which, by the way, is just two glasses of wine!), you probably only have 300 calories left for dinner. You don't have to lock yourself in—you can still live large, just eat small. Strategize!

Urban Skinny: *Losing weight is work—if it weren't, nobody would be overweight.*

Now that you know how many calories you get in a day and how to distribute them, let's start spending. But first, let's do a quick comparison.

Here's a non–Urban Skinny day versus an Urban Skinny day:

Non–Urban Skinny Day

Breakfast: bagel, cream cheese,
medium whole-milk latte...................................... (900 calories)

Lunch: the average pre-made chicken Caesar
salad with chicken, dressing, croutons, and
Parmesan cheese.. (900 calories)

Snack: slice of office birthday cake .... (400 calories)

Dinner: martini, half a bottle of wine, crusty roll,
pecan-crusted salmon with wasabi mashed potatoes
and asparagus, half a molten chocolate cake .... (1550 calories)

Total: .... 3800 calories

If you're a typical 5'4" woman, you just consumed more than two days' worth of food in one day!

Urban Skinny Day

Breakfast: 3 egg whites with one slice cheese and tomato on dry whole-wheat toast, small skim cappuccino .... (400 calories)

Lunch: slice of pizza with cheese and veggies........... (500 calories)

Snack: apple, 15 almonds.. (200 calories)

Dinner: 1 glass of wine, arugula salad with the dressing on the side, grilled halibut, steamed veggies, and a *bite* of dessert .... (550 calories)

Total: .... 1650 calories

The Urban Skinny day is half the calories of the previous menu. Look how much you can eat and stay within your budget! Added bonus: You also had calcium, fruit, veggies, protein, heart-healthy omega-3, and whole grains.

URBAN INSIGHT: If you flew to London you'd take the time to learn the exchange rate on the dollar so you wouldn't blow too much money at Harrods. Why not learn what your food is costing you in added pounds? In order to spend, you need to know the price of things—shopping and eating have the same principles. Remember to check labels and go online before you hit a chain restaurant; they all post calorie counts on their Web sites. Make sure you're counting calories and staying within your budget.

Urban Skinny: *Cappuccinos have fewer calories than lattes do (less milk, more foam)—especially if you order one with skim milk!*

Urban Skinny Quick Calorie Counter

Here's a quick reference guide that should help you learn calorie counting. You can print a copy out at UrbanSkinny.com. Keep it on your desk
and on the fridge for fast reference.

Fruit 75–100 calories (the size of a tennis ball)
- 1 banana
- 1 apple/pear
- 4 dried apricots
- 1 cup melon/berries
- 3 tablespoons raisins or dried cranberries
- 6 ounces fruit juice
- 4 dried prunes

Vegetables freebies
If sautéed add 50–100 calories

Starch 100 calories (1 ounce dry)
- 1 small potato/yam
- 1 slice bread
- ½ cup cooked pasta
- ½ cup cooked rice
- ½ cup cooked grains

Urban Myth: *Carbs are evil.*

Urban Skinny: *Anybody who stays lean long-term eats things
like sweet potatoes, bananas, pasta, and sandwiches. Try to eat
whole grains, but it's all about portion control. A half of a whole-
wheat bagel is about 250 calories.*

- ☐ ½ cup cooked peas
- ☐ ½ cup cooked corn
- ☐ ½ cup cooked edamame, shelled
- ☐ ½ cup cooked beans, like lentils or chickpeas
- ☐ 1 ounce dry cereal (read labels, servings vary)
- ☐ 1 small dinner roll
- ☐ 2 flatbreads
- ☐ 7 saltines
- ☐ 1 English muffin (120–140 calories)
- ☐ ½ flour tortilla (120 calories)
- ☐ 1 pita (140 calories)

Protein 3 ounces cooked, 21 grams of protein (size of palm of hand or deck of cards)

Leanest: 100 calories, 0–3 grams of fat
- ☐ white turkey
- ☐ white-meat chicken
- ☐ white fish
- ☐ shellfish
- ☐ 6 egg whites
- ☐ ¾ cup cottage cheese with 0–1% fat

Lean: 165 calories, 9 grams of fat
- ☐ salmon/Chilean sea bass
- ☐ dark-meat chicken or turkey (no skin)
- ☐ sirloin, 90–92% lean
- ☐ pork tenderloin
- ☐ veal chop
- ☐ lamb chop
- ☐ ground turkey

Medium: 225 calories, 15 grams of fat
- ☐ 3 eggs
- ☐ fried chicken
- ☐ veal scaloppine
- ☐ ground chicken
- ☐ filet mignon
- ☐ a burger from a diner
- ☐ short ribs
- ☐ brisket

Fattiest: 300 calories, 30 grams of fat
- ☐ sausage
- ☐ cheese
- ☐ spare ribs
- ☐ hot dogs
- ☐ salami

Fat 100 calories (8–10 grams)
- ☐ 1 tablespoon oil (120 calories)
- ☐ 1 tablespoon peanut butter, mayo, or butter (100 calories)
- ☐ 2 tablespoons nuts (100 calories [10 calories per nut])
- ☐ 2 tablespoons vinaigrette (100 calories)
- ☐ 2 strips bacon (100 calories)
- ☐ ¼ avocado (100 calories)

Alcohol
- ☐ 6 ounces wine (150 calories)
- ☐ 1 light beer (100 calories)
- ☐ 1 ounce vodka with club soda (100 calories)

☐ 1 ounce vodka with tonic (150 calories)

☐ 1 martini or cosmo (200 calories)

Sushi

☐ 1 roll (6 pieces) (240 calories)

☐ 1 California roll (150 calories)

☐ 1 piece of sushi (50 calories)

☐ 1 piece of sashimi (25–35 calories)

Extras

☐ protein in a gravy/sauce (add 200–300 calories)

☐ protein pan-seared/a little shiny (add 100 calories)

☐ slice of fruit pie (350 calories)

☐ 2-inch cookie (75 calories)

☐ black-and-white cookie (400 calories)

☐ New York bagel (450 calories [550 calories with cream cheese])

☐ small skim cappuccino (80 calories)

☐ 1 large muffin (500–600 calories)

☐ slice of cheese pizza, blotted to get rid of grease, veggies only (400–500 calories)

URBAN INSIGHT: Think like a New Yorker: Manage your weight like it's your job.

In the beginning make it easy on yourself and start by counting calories by the hundreds. Guys love this method: They take a list of 100-calorie foods and start plugging away until they get the hang of counting. Here's a starter list:

100-Calorie Foods to Get You through the Day

1 piece of fruit
1 cup of fruit
5 dried apricots
5 prunes
6 ounces fruit juice
1 cup Cheerios
1 cup Special K
1 packet plain oatmeal
1 packet Quaker Lower Sugar
  instant oatmeal
1 slice bread
¼ New York bagel
1 small baked potato
100-calorie snack bags
  (Nabisco)
1 Thomas' 100-calorie English
  muffin
½ cup cooked pasta, rice, or
  beans
3 ounces chicken or turkey
  (white meat, no skin)
3 ounces shellfish or white fish
  (size of a deck of cards)
2 pieces sushi
4 pieces sashimi
1 sushi roll with 6 pieces
  (no rice)
3 shumai (Chinese dumplings)
1 tablespoon mayo
1 tablespoon oil
1 tablespoon peanut butter
2 tablespoons vinaigrette
  dressing
10 large olives

10 almonds or walnuts
20 peanuts or pistachios
1 ounce cheese
1 string cheese
100-calorie bag of almonds
  (Blue Diamond)
2 Oreos
½ cup light ice cream
2 Hershey Miniatures
4 Hershey's Kisses
1 fun-size candy bar
5 Twizzlers
10 peanut M&M's
20 chocolate M&M's
8–10 ounces skim or low-fat
  milk
6 ounces plain yogurt
6 egg whites
1 cup applesauce (no sugar)
4 ounces wine
12 ounces light beer
1 shot alcohol
8 ounces soda
1 small skim latte
1 medium skim cappuccino
1 tall Caffé Frappuccino Light
  (any flavor)
4-ounce container fat-free
  pudding
4-ounce container sugar-free
  pudding (60–70 calories)
4-ounce container fat-free or
  0–1% fat cottage cheese

Vitamins and Supplements

Vitamins and supplements are like insurance. They cover your butt in case you don't get all of the nutrients you need from the food you eat. They don't replace food; they supplement it. Women: Take a women's formula multivitamin daily, and a calcium citrate supplement, such as Citracal. Calcium citrate is more efficiently absorbed than the form of calcium found in Tums and Viactiv. Men: Take a multivitamin daily. There's no need for mega or ultra formula options. More isn't better; you just need 100 percent of your daily nutrients in whatever you take. Omega-3 supplements have been said to reduce your risk of heart disease—not a must, but a good idea.

Urban Recap

Learn what food costs you in calories so you can spend wisely without going over your budget.

Urban Myth: *Always make your appetizer a salad.*

Urban Skinny: *Ceviche, shrimp cocktail, and lump crab are great options, too. If you want a salad before an entrée, make it a vegetable salad only. If you get the beet and cheese or tomato and mozzarella or anything with nuts, you need to make that your entire meal—not your starter.*

Up Next

All this talk of fat and protein may be as confusing as trying to figure out why the guy you went out with three times (and had fun with!) didn't call back. Here's the thing: You'll figure out the nutritional stuff sooner—it's much easier to understand. But if it still confuses you, as with everything else in New York and other big cities, you can hire someone to do the work for you. Urban Skinny is your hire. In the next chapter, if your brain hurts too much from everything else, let us do the work for you. No thinking required. If you just want to eat from the lists you'll see next, do it and don't deviate; stay the course. You'll have purged Mr. Wrong from your brain and left lots of room to concentrate on looking hot.

> **Urban Myth:** *Fat makes you fat.*
>
> **Urban Skinny:** *Fat, fortunately, is great. It actually helps you lose weight because it makes meals more satisfying and keeps you full longer. Include a little fat in every meal. A tablespoon of olive oil or a tablespoon of peanut butter is only about 100 calories. Why eat dry toast or salad with just vinegar if you don't have to?*

CHAPTER 3

Stay the Course—
Stick to the Plan

Gillian, 5'7", 44 years old, super social, ate anything she wanted until her late thirties without weight ramifications.

Urban Challenge
Gillian was not a major exerciser except for a bit of yoga. She drank her wine and ate her red meat, until all of a sudden it caught up to her out of nowhere. When she had a child she gained 20 pounds and couldn't shake them.

Urban Surprise
Gillian packaged her weight very well. She weighed 165 pounds—but it didn't show.

Urban Insight
Gillian thought she could lose the weight through exercise alone and went to see a trainer. But even though she worked out like crazy and did several 40-minute cardio blasts a week, her weight didn't budge.

After keeping a food log, Gillian realized that although she was very motivated with her workouts, she simply ate too much—almost 2000 calories a day. Even during Urban Skinny she still enjoyed one glass of *wine at dinner and even two or three glasses of wine on a girls' night out. But overall, she shaved 300 calories a day off her intake and in a month lost 10 pounds. She was very busy and goal oriented, and simply wanted to know what to eat without giving it all too much thought, so she just followed Urban Skinny. Gillian circled her picks on the Urban Skinny chart—no thought required. She kept it simple, with no starch and no improvisations. She ate out a lot and just stuck to simple steak and veggie, fish and veggie, or chicken and veggie options. She got her weight down to around 140 pounds.*

Eliminate the Guesswork

We've given you some tools—how many calories you can eat, how to space them out, and how to track them. We gave you some general lists so you know what you're eating, but until you really learn calories the same way you learned to talk your way into an invite-only party, it can be tough. Learning what to actually eat each meal and each day takes some time. Eventually it will be second nature, but until it is, stick to the lists below as much as possible. Some people never deviate and just follow this list forever. At least for now, and until you decide how you're going to play it long-term, *Urban Skinny* will do the work for you—especially helpful if your mind is on overload.

> Avoid enriched flour by sticking to 100% whole wheat. White flour is stripped of all the good things, like fiber, so read your labels. Even if it is "whole grain," check the ingredient list: If it says "enriched flour," put it back.

Here's how: Pick one of the meal plans offered here and stick to it. If you do it for even just a week or two, you'll get a great handle on how to count calories. Pick a meal from each category based on your daily caloric intake.

Here are some sample meal plans for each calorie group. For things like cereal or yogurt, if you want to switch out the brand, read the label and match the calories. Always buy 100% whole-wheat bread, bagels, English muffins, and pita.

1200 CALORIES: Choose One Selection for Each Meal

Breakfast Selections
300 calories

Made at home:

PB: 1 slice whole-wheat bread topped with 1 tablespoon peanut or nut butter and 1 small banana

Eggs: 4-egg-white omelet made with veggies and 1 ounce cheese, served with 1 whole-wheat English muffin

Yogurt: 6 ounces Fage Total 0% yogurt topped with 2 tablespoons chopped nuts, ½ cup berries, and ½ cup Fiber One cereal

Oatmeal: 1 packet Kashi Go Lean oatmeal made with skim milk and topped with 2 tablespoons chopped/slivered almonds/walnuts

Cereal: 1 cup Kashi Go Lean Crunch! Honey Almond Flax cereal topped with ¾ cup skim milk and ½ banana

Out of the house:

Deli: 3 egg whites with 1 slice cheese on 2 slices whole-wheat bread

On the go: 1 Balance or ZonePerfect bar with 1 piece or 1 cup of fruit

Parfait: 8-ounce yogurt parfait

Omelet: Egg-white omelet with veggies and cheese (diner)

Lunch Selections
300–400 calories

Made at home:

Sandwich: 3 ounces (about 3 slices) turkey breast and 1 ounce (2 thin slices) cheese or ¼ avocado on a whole-wheat pita with 1 cup chopped veggies

Tuna: 3 ounces tuna made with 2 tablespoons light mayo or 1 tablespoon regular mayo served with 1 whole-wheat English muffin and 1 cup chopped veggies

Entrée: Amy's, Lean Cuisine, or Weight Watchers Smart Ones frozen meal (minimum 300 calories)

Out of the house:

Salad: Large mixed salad topped with 1 "tong" each of chicken and chickpeas, black beans, or kidney beans, with 2 ounces vinaigrette dressing

Wrap: ½ wrap or gourmet sandwich with 1 cup chopped veggies

Soup: 12 ounces turkey chili

Afternoon Snack Selections
150–200 calories

20–25 almonds

10–15 almonds and 1 small piece of fruit

1 Balance Gold or ZonePerfect bar

1 small apple and 1 tablespoon peanut or nut butter

1 string cheese (80 calories) and 1 piece of fruit

Up to 200 calories of anything (i.e., answer your cravings)

Dinner Selections
400–450 calories

All meals need to include the following

Lean meat: 6 ounces grilled white fish, shellfish, or white-meat chicken or 4 ounces meat or fatty fish

Vegetables: Steamed veggies (unlimited)

Salad: Mixed vegetable salad with 2 tablespoons vinagrette dressing (100 calories)

Starch: ½ cup cooked starch (opt for whole grains!)

1300 CALORIES: Choose One Selection for Each Meal

Breakfast Selections

300–350 calories

Made at home:

PB: 1 slice whole-wheat bread topped with 1½ tablespoons peanut or nut butter and 1 small banana

Eggs: 4-egg-white omelet made with veggies and 1 ounce cheese served with 1 whole-wheat English muffin

Yogurt: 6 ounces Fage Total 0% yogurt topped with 2 tablespoons chopped nuts, 3 tablespoons dried berries, and ½ cup Fiber One cereal

Oatmeal: 1 packet Kashi Go Lean oatmeal made with skim milk and topped with 2 tablespoons chopped/slivered almonds/walnuts and ½ banana

Cereal: 1 cup Kashi Go Lean Crunch! Honey Almond Flax cereal topped with ¾ cup skim milk and ½ banana

Out of the house:

Deli: 3 egg whites with 1 slice cheese on 2 slices whole-wheat bread

On the go: 1 Balance or ZonePerfect bar with 1 piece or 1 cup of fruit

Parfait: 8-ounce yogurt parfait

Omelet: Egg-white omelet with veggies and cheese (diner)

Lunch Selections

350–400 calories

Made at home:

Sandwich: 3 ounces (about 3 slices) turkey breast and 1 ounce (2 thin slices) cheese and 1 tablespoon light mayo on a whole-wheat pita with 1 cup chopped veggies

Tuna: 3 ounces tuna made with 2 tablespoons light mayo or 1 tablespoon regular mayo served with 1 whole-wheat English muffin and 1 cup chopped veggies

Entrée: Amy's, Lean Cuisine, or Weight Watchers Smart Ones frozen meal (minimum 350–400 calories; if less than 300, add 1 piece of fruit)

Out of the house:

Salad: Large mixed salad topped with 1 "tong" each of chicken and chickpeas, black or kidney beans, with 2 tablespoons vinaigrette dressing

Wrap: ½ wrap or gourmet sandwich with 1 cup chopped veggies

Soup: 12 ounces turkey chili, small piece of fruit

Afternoon Snack Selections

150–200 calories

20–25 almonds

10–15 almonds and 1 small piece of fruit

1 Balance Gold or ZonePerfect bar

1 small apple and 1 tablespoon peanut or nut butter

1 string cheese (80 calories) and 1 piece of fruit

Up to 200 calories of anything (i.e., answer your cravings)

Dinner Selections

400–450 calories

All meals need to include the following

Lean meat: 6 ounces grilled white fish, shellfish, or white-meat chicken or 4 ounces meat or fatty fish

Vegetables: Steamed veggies (unlimited)

Salad: Mixed vegetable salad with 2 tablespoons vinaigrette dressing (100 calories)

Starch: ½ cup cooked starch (opt for whole grains!)

1400 CALORIES: Choose One Selection for Each Meal

Breakfast Selections

350 calories

Made at home:

PB: 1 slice whole-wheat bread topped with 1½ tablespoons peanut or nut butter and 1 small banana

Eggs: 5-egg-white omelet made with veggies and 1 ounce cheese served with 1 whole-wheat English muffin

Yogurt: 6 ounces Fage Total 0% yogurt topped with 2 tablespoons chopped nuts, 3 tablespoons dried berries, and ½ cup Fiber One cereal

Oatmeal: 1 packet Kashi Go Lean oatmeal made with skim milk and topped with 2 tablespoons chopped/slivered almonds/walnuts and ½ banana

Cereal: 1 cup Kashi Go Lean Crunch! Honey Almond Flax cereal topped with ¾ cup skim milk and ½ banana

Out of the house:

Deli: 3 egg whites with 1 slice cheese on 2 slices whole-wheat bread

On the go: 1 Balance or ZonePerfect bar with 6 ounces nonfat or low-fat yogurt

Parfait: 8-ounce yogurt parfait

Omelet: Egg-white omelet with veggies and cheese, 6 ounces OJ (diner)

Lunch Selections

400 calories

Made at home:

Sandwich: 3 ounces (about 3 slices) turkey breast and 1 ounce (2 thin slices) cheese and 1 tablespoon light mayo on a whole-wheat pita with 1 cup chopped veggies

Tuna: 3 ounces tuna made with 2 tablespoons light mayo or 1 tablespoon regular mayo served with 1 whole-wheat English muffin and ½ cup berries/fruit

Entrée: Amy's, Lean Cuisine, or Weight Watchers Smart Ones frozen meal (minimum 350–400 calories; if less than 300, add 1 piece of fruit)

Out of the house:

Salad: Large mixed salad topped with 1 "tong" each of chicken, orange wedges, and chickpeas, black beans or kidney beans, with 2 ounces vinaigrette dressing

Wrap: ½ wrap or gourmet sandwich with 8 ounces gazpacho or other veggie-only soup

Soup: 16 ounces turkey chili

Pizza: 1 slice pizza topped with veggies (once a week only)

Afternoon Snack Selections

200 calories

20–25 almonds

10–15 almonds and 1 small piece of fruit

1 Balance Gold or ZonePerfect bar

1 apple and 1 tablespoon peanut or nut butter

1 string cheese (80 calories) and 1 piece of fruit

Up to 200 calories of anything (i.e., answer your cravings)

Dinner Selections

400–500 calories

All meals need to include the following

Lean meat: 6 ounces grilled white fish, shellfish, or white-meat chicken or 4–5 ounces meat or fatty fish

Vegetables: Steamed veggies (unlimited)

Salad: Mixed vegetable salad with 2 tablespoons vinaigrette dressing (100 calories)

Starch: ½ cup cooked starch (opt for whole grains!)

1500 CALORIES: Choose One Selection for Each Meal

Breakfast Selections

350–400 calories

Made at home:

PB: 1 slice whole-wheat bread topped with 1½ tablespoons peanut or nut butter and 1 large banana

Eggs: 4-egg-white omelet made with veggies and 1 ounce cheese served with 1 whole-wheat English muffin and 1 cup berries

Yogurt: 6 ounces Fage Total 0% yogurt topped with 2 tablespoons chopped nuts, ¼ cup dried berries, and ½ cup Fiber One cereal

Oatmeal: 1 packet Kashi Go Lean oatmeal made with skim milk and topped with 2 tablespoons chopped/slivered almonds/walnuts and ½ banana

Cereal: 1 cup Kashi Go Lean Crunch! cereal topped with ¾ cup skim milk, ½ banana, and 2 tablespoons chopped/slivered almonds

Out of the house:

Deli: 3 egg whites with 1 slice cheese on 2 slices whole-wheat bread and 1 small piece of fruit

On the go: 1 Balance or ZonePerfect bar with 6 ounces Fage Total yogurt and 1 piece or 1 cup of fruit

Parfait: 8-ounce yogurt parfait topped with 2 tablespoons chopped nuts

Omelet: Egg-white omelet with veggies and cheese and 1 slice whole-wheat toast (diner)

Lunch Selections

400–450 calories

Made at home:

Sandwich: 3 ounces (about 3 slices) turkey breast and 1 ounce (2 thin slices) cheese and 1 tablespoon light mayo on a whole-wheat pita with 1 cup chopped veggies

Tuna: 3 ounces tuna made with 2 tablespoons light mayo or 1 tablespoon regular mayo served with 1 whole-wheat English muffin and 1 piece or 1 cup of fruit

Entrée: Amy's, Lean Cuisine, or Weight Watchers Smart Ones frozen meal (minimum 300–400 calories; if less than 300, add side salad with 2 tablespoons oil-based dressing—100 calories)

Out of the house:

Salad: Large mixed salad topped with 1 "tong" each of chicken, orange wedges, and chickpeas, black beans, or kidney beans, with 2 ounces vinaigrette dressing

Wrap: ½ wrap or gourmet sandwich with 8 ounces bean soup

Soup: 16 ounces turkey chili

Pizza: 1 slice pizza topped with veggies (only once a week)

Afternoon Snack Selections

200 calories

20–25 almonds

10–15 almonds and 1 small piece of fruit

1 Balance Gold or ZonePerfect bar

1 apple and 1 tablespoon peanut or nut butter

1 string cheese (80 calories) and 1 piece of fruit

Up to 200 calories of anything (i.e., answer your cravings)

Dinner Selections

500 calories

All meals need to include the following

Lean meat: 6 ounces grilled white fish, shellfish, or white-meat chicken or 5 ounces meat or fatty fish

Vegetables: Steamed veggies (unlimited)

Salad: Mixed vegetable salad with 2 tablespoons vinaigrette dressing (100 calories)

Starch: ¾ cup cooked starch (opt for whole grains!)

1600 CALORIES: Choose One Selection for Each Meal

Breakfast Selections
400 calories
Made at home:

PB: 1 whole-wheat English muffin topped with 1½ tablespoons peanut or nut butter and 1 large banana

Eggs: 5-egg-white omelet made with veggies and 1 ounce cheese served with 1 whole-wheat English muffin and 1 cup berries

Yogurt: 6 ounces Fage Total 0% yogurt topped with 2 ounces (½ cup) Bear Naked granola and ½ cup fresh berries

Oatmeal: 1 packet Kashi Go Lean oatmeal made with skim milk and topped with 2 tablespoons chopped/slivered almonds/walnuts and 3 tablespoons dried berries

Cereal: 1 cup Kashi Go Lean Crunch! cereal topped with ¾ cup skim milk, ½ banana, and 2 tablespoons chopped/slivered almonds

Out of the house:

Deli: 3 egg whites with 1 slice cheese on 2 slices whole-wheat bread and 1 small piece of fruit

On the go: 1 Balance or ZonePerfect bar with 6 ounces Fage Total yogurt and 1 piece or 1 cup of fruit

Parfait: 8-ounce yogurt parfait topped with 2 tablespoons chopped nuts

Omelet: Egg-white omelet with veggies and cheese and 1 slice whole-wheat toast (diner)

Lunch Selections
400–500 calories
Made at home:

Sandwich: 4 ounces (about 4 slices) turkey breast and 1 ounce (2 thin slices) cheese and 1 tablespoon light mayo on a whole-wheat pita with 1 cup chopped veggies

Tuna: 3 ounces tuna made with 2 tablespoons light mayo or 1 tablespoon regular mayo on a whole-wheat pita with 1 piece or 1 cup of fruit

Entrée: Amy's, Lean Cuisine, or Weight Watchers Smart Ones frozen meal (minimum 300 calories; if less than 300, add side salad with 3 tablespoons vinaigrette dressing—150 calories)

Out of the house:

Salad: Large mixed salad topped with 1 "tong" each of chicken, avocado, and chickpeas, black beans, or kidney beans, with 2 ounces vinaigrette dressing

Wrap: ½ wrap or gourmet sandwich with 8 ounces bean soup

Soup: 16 ounces turkey chili or seafood gumbo and 1 small piece of fruit

Pizza: 1 slice pizza topped with veggies (once a week only)

Afternoon Snack Selections

200 calories

20–25 almonds

10–15 almonds and 1 small piece of fruit

1 Balance Gold or ZonePerfect bar

1 apple and 1 tablespoon peanut or nut butter

1 string cheese (80 calories) and 1 piece of fruit

Up to 200 calories of anything (i.e., answer your cravings)

Dinner Selections

500–600 calories

All meals need to include the following

Lean meat: 6 ounces grilled white fish, shellfish, or white-meat chicken or 4 ounces meat or fatty fish

Vegetables: Steamed veggies (unlimited)

Salad: Mixed vegetable salad with 2 tablespoons vinaigrette dressing (100 calories)

Starch: 1 cup cooked starch (opt for whole grains!)

1700 CALORIES: Choose One Selection for Each Meal

Breakfast Selections

400–450 calories

Made at home:

PB: 2 slices whole-wheat bread topped with 2 tablespoons peanut or nut butter and 1 large banana

Eggs: 6-egg-white omelet made with veggies and 1 ounce cheese served with 2 slices whole-wheat toast and 1 cup berries or 1 piece of fruit

Yogurt: 6 ounces Fage Total 0% yogurt topped with 2 ounces (½ cup) Bear Naked granola and 3 tablespoons dried berries

Oatmeal: 2 packets Kashi Go Lean oatmeal made with half water and half skim milk and topped with 2 tablespoons chopped/slivered almonds/walnuts

Cereal: 1 cup Kashi Go Lean Crunch! cereal with ¾ cup skim milk, ½ banana, and 2 tablespoons chopped/slivered almonds

Out of the house:

Deli: 4 egg whites with 1 slice cheese on 2 slices whole-wheat bread and 1 piece or 1 cup of fruit

On the go: 1 Clif or Greens+ bar with 5 ounces Fage Total yogurt and 1 piece or 1 cup of fruit

Parfait: 8-ounce yogurt parfait topped with 3 tablespoons chopped nuts

Omelet: Egg-white omelet with veggies and cheese and 2 slices whole-wheat toast (diner)

Lunch Selections

500 calories

Made at home:

Sandwich: 4 ounces (about 4 slices) turkey breast and 1 ounce (2 thin slices) cheese and 1 tablespoon light mayo on a whole-wheat pita with 1 piece of fruit

Tuna: 6 ounces tuna made with 2 tablespoons light mayo or 1 tablespoon regular mayo on 2 slices whole-wheat bread and 1 cup fruit

Entrée: Amy's, Lean Cuisine, or Weight Watchers Smart Ones frozen meal (300–400 calories; if less than 300, add side salad with 3 tablespoons vinaigrette dressing—150 calories)

Out of the house:

Salad: Large mixed salad topped with 1 "tong" each of chicken, egg whites, avocado, and chickpeas, black beans, or kidney beans, with 2 ounces vinaigrette dressing

Wrap: ½ wrap or gourmet sandwich with 8 ounces bean soup or small side salad with 2 tablespoons vinaigrette dressing

Soup: 16 ounces turkey chili and 1 small piece of fruit

Pizza: 1 slice pizza topped with veggies

Afternoon Snack Selections

200–250 calories

30–35 almonds

2-ounce bag mixed nuts and dried fruit

20 almonds and 1 small piece of fruit

1 Balance Gold or ZonePerfect bar

1 apple and 1½ tablespoons peanut or nut butter

2 string cheeses (80 calories each) and 1 piece of fruit

Up to 250 calories of anything (i.e., answer your cravings)

Dinner Selections

550–600 calories

All meals need to include the following

Lean meat: 6 ounces grilled white fish, shellfish, or white-meat chicken or 6 ounces meat or fatty fish

Vegetables: Steamed veggies cooked with 1 tablespoon olive oil

Salad: Mixed vegetable salad with 3 tablespoons vinaigrette dressing (150 calories)

Starch: 1 cup cooked starch (opt for whole grains!)

1800 CALORIES: Choose One Selection for Each Meal

Breakfast Selections
450 calories

Made at home:

PB: 2 slices whole-wheat bread topped with 2 tablespoons peanut or nut butter and 1 large banana

Eggs: 6-egg-white omelet made with veggies and 1 ounce cheese served with 2 slices whole-wheat toast and 1 cup berries or 1 piece of fruit

Yogurt: 6 ounces Fage Total 0% yogurt topped with 2 ounces (½ cup) Bear Naked granola and 3 tablespoons dried berries

Oatmeal: 2 packets Kashi Go Lean oatmeal made with half water and half skim milk and topped with 2 tablespoons chopped/slivered almonds/walnuts

Cereal: 1 cup Kashi Go Lean Crunch! cereal topped with ¾ cup skim milk, 1 banana, and 2 tablespoons chopped/slivered almonds

Out of the house:

Deli: 4 egg whites with 2 slices cheese on 2 slices whole-wheat bread with 1 piece or 1 cup of fruit

On the go: 1 Clif or Greens+ bar with 6 ounces Fage Total yogurt and 1 piece or 1 cup of fruit

Parfait: 8-ounce yogurt parfait topped with 3 tablespoons chopped nuts

Omelet: Egg-white omelet with veggies and cheese and 2 slices whole-wheat toast (diner)

Lunch Selections
500–550 calories

Made at home:

Sandwich: 4 ounces (about 4 slices) turkey breast and 1 ounce (2 thin slices) cheese and smear of mayo on a whole-wheat pita with 1 piece of fruit

Tuna: 6 ounces tuna made with 2 tablespoons light mayo or 1 tablespoon regular mayo on 2 slices whole-wheat bread with 1 cup fruit

Entrée: Amy's, Lean Cuisine, or Weight Watchers Smart Ones frozen meal (300–400 calories) and side salad with 3 tablespoons vinaigrette dressing (150 calories)

Out of the house:

Salad: Large mixed salad topped with 1 "tong" each of chicken, egg whites, avocado, and chickpeas, black beans, or kidney beans, with 2 ounces vinaigrette dressing

Wrap: ½ wrap or gourmet sandwich with 8 ounces bean soup or small side salad with 2 tablespoons vinaigrette dressing

Soup: 16 ounces turkey chili and 1 small piece of fruit

Pizza: 1 slice pizza topped with veggies

Afternoon Snack Selections

200–250 calories

30–35 almonds

2-ounce bag mixed nuts and dried fruit

20 almonds and 1 small piece of fruit

1 Balance Bar Gold or Zone bar

1 apple and 1½ tablespoons peanut or nut butter

2 string cheeses (80 calories each) and 1 piece of fruit

Up to 250 calories of anything (i.e., answer your cravings)

Dinner Selections

600–650 calories

All meals need to include the following

Lean meat: 6 ounces grilled white fish, shellfish, or white-meat chicken or 6 ounces meat or fatty fish

Vegetables: Steamed veggies cooked with 1 tablespoon olive oil

Salad: Mixed vegetable salad with 3 tablespoons vinaigrette dressing (150 calories)

Starch: 1 cup cooked starch (opt for whole grains!)

1900 CALORIES: Choose One Selection for Each Meal

Breakfast Selections
450–500 calories

Made at home:

PB: 2 slices whole-wheat bread topped with 2 tablespoons peanut or nut butter and 1 large banana

Eggs: 6-egg-white omelet made with veggies and 1 ounce cheese served with 2 slices whole-wheat toast and 1 cup berries or 1 piece of fruit

Yogurt: 6 ounces Fage Total 0% yogurt topped with 2 ounces (½ cup) Bear Naked granola and 3 tablespoons dried berries

Oatmeal: 2 packets Kashi Go Lean oatmeal made with half water and half skim milk and topped with 2 tablespoons chopped/slivered almonds/walnuts

Cereal: 1½ cups Kashi Go Lean Crunch! cereal topped with 1 cup skim milk, ½ banana, and 2 tablespoons chopped/slivered almonds

Out of the house:

Deli: 4 egg whites with 2 slices cheese on 2 slices whole-wheat bread and 1 piece or 1 cup of fruit

On the go: 1 Clif or Greens+ bar with 6 ounces Fage Total yogurt and 1 large piece or 1½ cups of fruit

Parfait: 8-ounce yogurt parfait topped with 3 tablespoons chopped nuts

Omelet: Egg-white omelet with veggies and cheese and 2 slices whole-wheat toast (diner)

Lunch Selections
550–600 calories

Made at home:

Sandwich: 4 ounces (about 4 slices) turkey breast and 1 ounce (2 thin slices) cheese and smear of mayo on whole-wheat bread with 1 piece of fruit

Tuna: 6 ounces tuna made with 2 tablespoons light mayo or 1 tablespoon regular mayo on 2 slices whole-wheat bread with 1 cup of fruit

Entrée: Amy's, Lean Cuisine, or Weight Watchers Smart Ones frozen meal (300–400 calories) and side salad with 4 tablespoons vinaigrette dressing (150 calories)

Out of the house:

Salad: Large mixed salad topped with 1 "tong" each of chicken, egg whites, avocado, and chickpeas, black beans, or kidney beans, with 2 ounces vinaigrette dressing

Wrap: ½ wrap or gourmet sandwich with 12 ounces bean soup or small side salad with 3 tablespoons vinaigrette dressing

Soup: 16 ounces turkey chili and side salad with 3 tablespoons vinaigrette dressing

Pizza: 1 slice pizza topped with vegetables and side salad with 2 tablespoons vinaigrette dressing

Afternoon Snack Selections

250 calories

35–40 almonds (1 large handful)

2-ounce bag mixed nuts and dried fruit

20 almonds and 1 large piece of fruit

1 Balance Gold or ZonePerfect bar and 1 small piece of fruit

1 apple and 1½ tablespoons peanut or nut butter

2 string cheeses (80 calories each) and 1 piece of fruit

Up to 250 calories of anything (i.e., answer your cravings

Dinner Selections

650–700 calories

All meals need to include the following

Lean meat: 6 ounces grilled white fish, shellfish, or white-meat chicken or 6 ounces meat or fatty fish

Vegetables: Steamed veggies cooked with 1 tablespoon olive oil

Salad: Mixed vegetable salad with 3 tablespoons vinaigrette dressing (150 calories)

Starch: 1 cup cooked starch (opt for whole grains!)

2000 CALORIES: Choose One Selection for Each Meal

Breakfast Selections

500 calories

Made at home:

PB: 2 slices whole-wheat bread topped with 2 tablespoons peanut or nut butter and 1 large banana

Eggs: 6-egg-white omelet made with veggies and 1 ounce cheese served with 2 slices whole-wheat toast and 1 cup berries or 1 piece of fruit

Yogurt: 6 ounces Fage Total 0% yogurt topped with 2 ounces (½ cup) Bear Naked granola and ¼ cup dried berries

Oatmeal: 2 packets Kashi Go Lean oatmeal made with skim milk and topped with 2 tablespoons chopped/slivered almonds/walnuts

Cereal: 1½ cups Kashi Go Lean Crunch! cereal with 1 cup skim milk, ½ banana, and 2 tablespoons chopped/slivered almonds

Out of the house:

Deli: 4 egg whites with 2 slices cheese on 2 slices whole-wheat bread and 1 piece or 1 cup of fruit

On the go: 1 Clif or Greens+ bar with 6 ounces Fage Total yogurt and 1 large piece or 1½ cups of fruit

Parfait: 16-ounce yogurt parfait

Omelet: Egg-white omelet with veggies and cheese and 2 slices whole-wheat toast (diner)

Lunch Selections

600 calories

Made at home:

Sandwich: 4 ounces (about 4 slices) turkey breast and 1 ounce (2 thin slices) cheese and smear of mayo on whole-wheat bread and side salad with 3 tablespoons vinaigrette dressing

Tuna: 6 ounces tuna made with 3 tablespoons light mayo or 1½ tablespoons regular mayo on 2 slices whole-wheat bread and 1 piece of fruit

Entrée: Amy's, Lean Cuisine, or Weight Watchers Smart Ones frozen meal (300–400 calories) and side salad with 3 tablespoons vinaigrette dressing (150 calories), 1 small piece of fruit

Out of the house:

Salad: Large mixed salad topped with 1 "tong" each chicken, egg whites, dried cranberries, avocado, and chickpeas, black beans, or kidney beans, with 2 ounces vinaigrette dressing

Wrap: ½ wrap or gourmet sandwich with 12 ounces bean soup or small side salad with 2 ounces vinaigrette dressing

Soup: 16 ounces turkey chili, side salad with 2 ounces vinaigrette dressing, and 1 piece of fruit

Pizza: 1 slice pizza topped with vegetables and side salad with 2 tablespoons vinaigrette dressing

Afternoon Snack Selections
250–300 calories

35–40 almonds (1 large handful)

2-ounce bag mixed nuts and dried fruit

20 almonds and 1 large piece of fruit

1 Balance Gold or ZonePerfect bar and 1 piece of fruit

1 large apple and 1½ tablespoons peanut or nut butter

2 string cheeses (80 calories each) and 1 piece of fruit

Up to 300 calories of anything (i.e., answer your cravings)

Dinner Selections
650–700 calories

All meals need to include the following

Lean meat: 6 ounces grilled white fish, shellfish, or white-meat chicken or 6 ounces meat or fatty fish

Vegetables: Steamed veggies cooked with 1 tablespoon olive oil

Salad: Mixed vegetable salad with 3 tablespoons vinaigrette dressing (150 calories)

Starch: 1 cup cooked starch (opt for whole grains!)

2200 CALORIES: Choose One Selection for Each Meal

Breakfast Selections

550 calories

Made at home:

PB: 2 slices whole-wheat bread topped with 2 tablespoons peanut or nut butter, 1 small banana, and 8 ounces skim milk

Eggs: 6-egg-white omelet made with veggies and 1½ ounces cheese served with 2 slices whole-wheat toast and 1 cup berries or 1 piece of fruit

Yogurt: 1½ cups Fage Total 0% yogurt topped with 2 ounces (½ cup) Bear Naked granola and ¾ cup dried berries

Oatmeal: 2 packets Kashi Go Lean oatmeal made with skim milk and topped with 3 tablespoons chopped/slivered almonds/walnuts

Cereal: 1½ cups Kashi Go Lean Crunch! cereal with 1 cup skim milk, ½ banana, and 2 tablespoons chopped/slivered almonds

Out of the house:

Deli: 4 egg whites with 2 slices cheese on a whole-wheat roll and 1 piece or 1 cup of fruit

On the go: 1 Detour bar with 6 ounces Fage Total yogurt and 1 large piece or 1½ cups of fruit

Parfait: 16-ounce yogurt parfait

Omelet: Egg-white omelet with veggies and cheese, 2 slices whole-wheat toast, and small bowl of fruit (diner)

Lunch Selections

650 calories

Made at home:

Sandwich: 4 ounces (about 4 slices) turkey breast and 1 ounce (2 thin slices) cheese and smear of mayo on whole-wheat bread and side salad with 4 tablespoons vinaigrette dressing

Tuna: 6 ounces tuna made with 3 tablespoons light mayo or 1½ tablespoons regular mayo on 2 slices whole-wheat bread with 2 pieces of fruit

Out of the house:

Salad: Large mixed salad topped with 1 "tong" each of chicken, dried cranberries, avocado, and chickpeas, black beans, or kidney beans, with 2 ounces vinaigrette dressing and 1 small whole-wheat roll

Wrap: ½ wrap or gourmet sandwich with 12 ounces bean soup or small side salad with 4 tablespoons vinaigrette dressing and 1 piece of fruit

Soup: 16 ounces turkey chili, side salad with 2 ounces vinaigrette dressing, and 1 piece of fruit

Pizza: 1 slice pizza topped with vegetables and side salad with 3 tablespoons vinaigrette dressing

Afternoon Snack Selections

300–350 calories

45–50 almonds (½ cup)

2-ounce bag mixed nuts and dried fruit and 6 ounces Fage Total yogurt

30 almonds and 1 large piece of fruit

1 Balance Gold, ZonePerfect, or Clif bar and 1 piece of fruit

2 slices whole-wheat bread topped with 1½ tablespoons peanut or nut butter

8- to 10-ounce fruit smoothie with protein powder

Up to 350 calories of anything (i.e., answer your cravings)

Dinner Selections

700–800 calories

All meals need to include the following

Lean meat: 6 ounces grilled white fish, shellfish, or white-meat chicken or 6 ounces meat or fatty fish

Vegetables: Steamed veggies cooked with 1 tablespoon olive oil

Salad: Mixed vegetable salad with 3 tablespoons vinaigrette dressing (150 calories)

Starch: 1½ cups cooked starch (opt for whole grains!)

URBAN INSIGHT: **With salad dressing, don't confuse ounces for table-spoons. Ask at lunch counters how much is in each little dressing container. The standard size is two ounces, which, for the record, is four tablespoons. So a two-ounce container of vinaigrette will cost you 200 calories; creamy dressing is 300 calories.**

Urban Recap

Stick to the simple picks for at least two weeks until you understand what you can eat; improvise only when it's something you can measure, like cereal.

Up Next

Even if you're keeping it simple, you can eat out. Some very basic restaurant rules will help you stay Urban Skinny, and some modifications during challenging social situations will help you stay on track. Nobody will even notice you're cutting back, but they'll notice how awesome you look in your new jeans.

CHAPTER 4

Ride in the
Fab Lane,
Not the
Flab Lane

John, 42 years old, Wall Street tycoon, lost 30 pounds following Urban Skinny.

Urban Challenge
John's work requires him to not only work all day in his office, but to entertain his clients after hours. He has to loosen them up over pre-dinner cocktails to seal the million-dollar deals. But steak dinner almost always follows the cocktails and that's where John got into calorie trouble. He used to be out four nights a week at a minimum and was making bad choices every time. He was big on anything fried or creamy—foods that were high in saturated fat and cholesterol were his true weakness. Veggies and fruit rarely made an appearance on John's plate any time of the day. He didn't mind fruit and veggies, but since that meant going to the store to actually buy them, it wasn't going to happen. For John, losing weight wasn't just about his pants not fitting—he'd also gotten a heads-up from his doctor about rising blood pressure.

Urban Surprise
John's success at work was largely due to his drive and ambition, so it comes as no surprise that no matter what time he got home at night,

he was in the pool at the crack of dawn. He trained hard at times for triathlons, until he hurt his back.

Urban Insight

Since John was so hard-core about work, when he decided to crack down and lose weight he took it on like it was his job. He now starts every meal with a salad. He switched to fish and chicken and only the occasional steak, and eased up on the booze, skipping the multiple martinis and switching to vodka and club soda for half the calories. He became the one who ordered at the bar so he could slip a plain soda with lime into the mix without anybody noticing. One major switch for John was scheduling lunch meetings instead of dinner meetings, so he could cut the booze and have a chance to eat a lighter dinner.

Urban Skinny to Go

Dining out is a rite of passage in big cities. In fact, some people get all three meals a day from a restaurant. What's the point of living in great culinary cities like New York and San Francisco if you can't embrace all of the incredible food they have to offer? Eating out or ordering in just about anything is what New Yorkers do. And every city has that great Chinese takeout place or a hot new must-see food stop. That's where Urban Skinny comes in. If you don't know how to cook, Urban Skinny is not going to teach you to cook. Instead it will educate you on how to eat out or order in and stay lean. Consider Urban Skinny your mini-Zagat guide, with a make-your-butt-look-great twist. Knowing how to order everything from drinks to snacks to dinner will boost your calorie-spending power.

Urban Myth: *Skipping meals saves calories.*

Urban Skinny: *You may think skipping a meal helps, but when you finally sit down to eat dinner, you'll probably be starving and hit that bread basket hard so you'll not only make up the difference but eat more.*

Urban Myth: *Sugar turns to fat. "Carbohydrate" is just a longer word for sugar.*

Urban Skinny: *People think bagels, pasta, and potatoes turn to fat. Everyone is on an anti-carb kick because they buy into this misconception. The bottom line is, anything eaten in excess adds extra pounds onto your body. There's no discriminating: The only thing that causes weight gain is extra calories. Carbs—which are sugar, it's true—don't add to your weight-loss challenge any more than any other nutrient does.*

Rules for Eating Out

You have to remember that going out to dinner can't always be a special occasion. If you live in a big city riddled with restaurants, eating out is simply a part of regular life. It's not an event—not every night, at least. Think of most meals out as just another meal except that someone else is cooking it for you. Look at it this way: If you're meeting up with some friends after work to grab a bite and it's a Tuesday (and you don't want your dinner to not only bite you in the ass, but become your ass), remember it's a Tuesday! Nothing overly exciting happens on a Tuesday. On Tuesday, eating out is just another meal, not an excuse to overeat. We tend to meet over food, but remember this: If you are seeing people you haven't seen for a while, getting the gossip, or whatever, make the meeting about enjoying your friends or your date, not the food. Take the focus off of the food!

Let's start with some basic eating-out rules that pertain to restaurant dining no matter which restaurant you're in. The same rules apply for every type of cuisine. The key to losing weight is eating consistently no matter which type of food you're eating—Indian, Chinese, or Italian. You need to follow the same rules you follow at home, but here are some tweaked ones for the restaurant connoisseur in you. Learn them and follow them—all the time.

You're going to get through the stress of beating the menu—with every meal you ever order from here on in. Simple, period, end of story! Here's the Skinny.

Rule Number 1:
Try to take control by choosing where you're eating.

We'll tell you how to order Mexican, but if you can steer the pick toward a place that's going to make your life a little easier by helping you beat temptation, that's a good thing. Don't feel like you have to go to a health food restaurant, but if it's a business dinner and you don't really care (it's just another work dinner), choosing something like Japanese or a seafood restaurant will help you out. Have you ever seen a bread basket at a Japanese restaurant?

Rule Number 2:
Research, research, research.

Before you even step foot in the restaurant you've chosen, know what you're going to order. How? C'mon, people, it's the Internet era! Go online. When you're sitting at work not doing your work, instead of ordering shoes from Zappos.com or reading your horoscope, check out the restaurant's menu. Decide ahead of time what you're going to order (we'll go through choices food by food later). You want to know going in what's available so you aren't influenced by other people's choices. If you have a game plan, you don't even have to look at the menu—don't even crack it; you'll already know what you're getting. Focus on the person or people you're with and let the food be the sidebar. Checking the menu online in advance gives you time to make a smart choice, avoiding the panic when the waiter arrives and forces your hand to the pick you probably should be skipping.

Rule Number 3:
Even if you don't always act like a lady, stick to the "ladies first" rule and order first.

Why? So that you're not influenced by other people's decisions. If you haven't ordered and someone else orders a gargantuan plate of gnocchi in a Gorgonzola cream sauce, you may think, hey, why not . . .

when in Rome. Here's the thing: You're not in freaking Rome. You don't get permission to fall just because someone else has. If staying strong means not sharing the fried calamari or the slab of foie gras, then that's what you gotta do. The bigger the group, the more you generally wind up eating, because your decision-making gets warped. Even if most people are dieting, it's likely they're doing it wrong. So stick to it . . . don't be a follower, be a leader—even at dinner—and don't jump on the food bandwagon.

Rule Number 4:
It's all about the salad.

Just because it's a "salad" doesn't make it your best option. You should always try to have a salad; it boosts your daily fruit and veggie intake. But choose your greens carefully. Don't get the ones with the nuts, cheese, cranberries, and crostini. Uh, yeah . . . just because the word "salad" is in the name, don't pretend it's okay. When you think salad, think vegetables. Ask for your dressing on the side. If you're going to put the effort in and order a salad instead of the fried spring roll, reap the reward of not having crammed an extra 300 calories into it. If you're not careful, your salad appetizer could be 400 calories or more. And that, my friends, is what we call an entrée.

> URBAN INSIGHT: Saladed out? Good apps to know: shrimp cocktail, lump crab, clams on the half shell, tuna or any seafood tartare, ceviche, or carpaccio, grilled vegetables (sans fromage and not slathered in oil), broth-based soup like consommé, or even gazpacho.

Rule Number 5:
Let's discuss the bread basket.

Okay, everyone's afraid of it, and with good reason. It's sitting there, you're starving, and it's usually good stuff. When it's willpower versus a nice hot fresh-from-the-oven, crispy-on-the-outside baguette, willpower never wins. Skill-power, however, has a fighting chance. Size it up: Is the bread the waiter just placed on the table inches from your nose worth the 100 calories? If a nice fresh-baked roll appeals to you more than the couscous that comes with your dinner, go for the one roll and enjoy. Operative word there being "one." If, however, you've been dying all day for the wasabi mashed potatoes you discovered come with your sea bass (when you did your research!), don't reach for the enemy. Don't. Don't do it. Keep the basket on the other side of the table. Strategize. You're not eating some crappy-ass dried-out roll just because it's there. Make a smart and satisfying choice.

Rule Number 6:
Your favorite restaurant is not likely to close down tomorrow.
You can go back any day. You don't have to eat everything on your plate or try everything on the menu every single time you visit. Restaurant portions are typically twice the size of what you eat at home, so if you want something, try it next time. This ain't your last supper, and you didn't get a heads-up on an upcoming famine in the big city.

Urban Myth: *Some foods are taboo.*

Urban Skinny: *Live a little. No foods are good or bad. The key is portion control and never overspending your calories. If you can't live without a donut, have one, but not three. Don't be greedy. A glazed Krispy Kreme donut is only about 200 calories.*

Rule Number 7:
You don't have to order an entrée.
A salad and an appetizer aren't such a bad way to go. Sometimes in a restaurant the appetizers look better than the entrées anyway. Also, when you get an appetizer as your main course, you don't get all the sides that sometimes come with the entrée, which leaves you wide open for that one roll you've been dreaming about. Apps are generally smaller portions, too.

Rule Number 8:

Opt for a protein that is grilled, broiled, blackened, or roasted in parchment or banana leaf.

Did you notice . . . fried isn't on the list? And sorry, "sauté" is just a fancy word for fried.

Rule Number 9:

When it comes to food, don't think big.

If you're in a panic because you're not sure of what's just been placed in front of you, or you didn't plan your order, or it wasn't what you expected, never fear. Just eat *less*. For example, if the fish you thought would arrive grilled looks fried and crusted, eat less of it. Smaller portions make smaller people.

When eating out, remember that restaurant portions are double and sometimes triple the amount you should be eating. You really have to learn to eyeball your portions and come as close as you can to knowing the difference between three ounces of steak and six ounces of steak. A deck of cards is three ounces and a woman's fist is a cup of rice. Guys, your fist is two cups. Also, always get your sauces and dressings on the side.

Rules are rules, but let's be honest, certain situations call for more specific strategy. The business dinner certainly isn't going to be treated the same way as the hot date or even the girls' night out. Here's the playbook for all sorts of tricky situations.

Date Night

You've got your hot new shoes. You had your hair professionally blown out but asked the stylist to make it look casual so you don't seem too eager. Mani-pedi? Check. You've done all the prep to make a good impression, but you don't want to be one of those girls who orders the air sandwich and a glass of water and just picks at her plate. Mr. Right's not going to appreciate paying 50 bucks for your Dover sole when you barely ate any of it. At the same time, we know you're not going to pig out and gorge anyway—how attractive would that be? But you do want to stick with the consistent eating habits you've been working on, even though you're sitting across from the hottest guy on the planet.

So what's a girl to do? He may want to share a bottle of wine. You don't want to say, "No, I can't. I'm on a diet." Instead, you say sure, and you simply sip slower than he does. Let him drink more than you (which, by the way, is good for all kinds of reasons). Sip, don't slug. Since you're having the wine, this is a good time to skip the bread basket.

Order the white fish—it's fewer calories and leaves you room for the alcohol. He may say, "Do you want to start with something?" You could be the one to say, "Let's share." Remember, a bite means just a bite. Take the bite of something. If he says he really wants you to try his short ribs (not a euphemism), take a bite. It won't tip you over the calorie edge, but he may think you're cool. If dessert enters into the picture, you could say you're full and ask to split something, or if he wants you to pick, order the berries or the sorbet. If you feel obligated, just have one or two bites if that mascarpone cheesecake ends up on the table somehow.

> The USDA suggests women have seven servings of fruit and veggies combined daily. Men should have nine. A starter salad should cover two of those.

Girls' Night Out

All right, you're waiting at the bar for that one friend who's always late, which means, of course, cocktails are in order. Cosmos and apple martinis are fashionable, yes. They may even match your nail polish. But what looks good in your hand doesn't look good on your butt. Lower-calorie drinks are key. A glass of champagne is a nice civilized choice; pink bubbles are in vogue these days. Or a vodka club with a splash of cranberry and lime is just about 100 calories, and you can ask for it in a martini glass if that makes you feel better. Even a glass of wine has

> Don't get too comfortable—wear your skinny jeans out so you don't stuff your face. You want to keep your pants buttoned throughout the entire meal, and a tight waist will be a good incentive.

fewer calories than the sweet martini-type drinks. And while flirting with the bartender might seem like a great idea, don't get too friendly, ladies—you don't need him making you an extra one on the house. If this is a long evening, have just one drink before you eat. That's it.

In general, girls share food. You could be the first to order, but you might be drawn into sharing lots of small plates. Don't be shy; if everyone's calling out picks, get yours in there. If you're eating tapas, include ceviche along with the

> **Bubbly is a calorie-saver at just 75 calories a glass—compared to more than 150 calories for a glass of wine. If your wallet isn't fat enough for the stuff from France, California-bottled Domaine Carneros by Taittinger makes award-winning sparkling wine that will knock your Jimmy Choo's off without making a big dent in your wallet.**

empanadas. Order chicken satay as well as the coconut shrimp. Even a slider is only 150 calories, so don't fret. Here's the danger though: If the entire meal consists of picking at small plates, you could lose track of what you order, and what goes in your mouth may add up more quickly than you think. Don't eat mindlessly. Think of the times when you sit in front of the TV and gulp back a bowl of popcorn before your favorite American Idol finishes his or her tune. Try not to eat everything that comes to the table; take a bite or two of each course and think about it as you eat it. And order your salad whenever you can.

A tip to cut down on the booze that's gonna be flowing: Order a big bottle of sparkling water and drink away. You might find you eat less because you're full, and you'll enjoy the sparkling water with lime like a refreshing cocktail. You'll finish the bottle, too, since you probably paid $15 for it, and you'll use the bubbles, not the bubbly, to quench your thirst. Convince the gang to skip dessert and hit the dance floor to burn some calories.

Business Dinner

Sometimes dining out is part of your job. You might be welcoming a new or prospective worker to the company or you're the one being welcomed. Lawyers do closing dinners, film and TV people have a wrap party, out-of-town clients need entertaining in every business, and those who work in finance know only half the work actually takes place in the office. Which brings us to the steak house—a place synonymous with closing the deal, almost a second office to those with that fat expense account. But remember, there's no such thing as a free meal. The company may pay for your dinner, but you'll pay in pounds in the end. (And we're not talking about the kind you traded at your currency desk today.) All the drink tips we've talked about still apply: Be the one who orders, choose Pellegrino or Perrier for the table, skip the martini during cocktail hour and save up for a glass of wine with dinner. If you're in a powerhouse profession, chances are good you're one of the few women at the table. If you are, remember you don't have to keep up with the men when it comes to food and booze; they eat more. Guys, you don't have to keep up with the other men either. Don't be a macho eater. Stick to your plan.

> **The USDA suggests one drink a day for women and two drinks a day for men. That's alcohol in moderation according to their dietary guidelines. That's one ounce of alcohol, four ounces of wine, or twelve ounces of beer.**

One good thing about a steak house: It's easy because the food is simple and consistent from place to place. But while it's basic, the portions can be a challenge because they are usually enormous. Some simple starters to stick with are the tomato onion salad, shrimp cocktail, a nice lump crab, and a salad—skip the lettuce wedge with the blue cheese and bacon and opt for the house green salad. It's sometimes hard (especially for guys) to order dressing on the side—you don't want to look like a wimp when you just closed a $17 million deal. The solution: Ask for the oil and vinegar; it's always served in little bottles on the side that you can control by pouring it on yourself. More vinegar than oil is a good idea.

On to the beef of the matter: The good thing about the steak house is the porterhouse for two. It might be twenty-four ounces, sliced up in two-to-three-ounce chunks. The "share" is the way to go. That's because the most you want to eat is about eight ounces, even as you watch the others at the table jam back an entire cow—a solid twenty-ounce rib eye is often the norm. You're *not* going to be that person. A standard portion of protein is three ounces, but we're being realistic; you're not getting out of there with just one bite. The petite filet is another option if nobody's ready to share; it's usually about eight ounces uncooked.

Don't be afraid: Ask the waiter about the ingredients and portion sizes.

Pull a *When Harry Met Sally* and make a special order if you need to.

But remember, red meat is high in saturated fat and cholesterol. A diet high in saturated fat has been shown to increase cholesterol levels, which are associated with an increased risk of cardiovascular disease and certain types of cancer. Keep in mind that sirloin has 55 calories an ounce and filet mignon has 75 calories an ounce. Some people mix that up. And if that's not macho enough for you (if you're a guy), order the surf and turf, which is usually a smaller cut of beef plus lobster or shrimp, which is half the calories of the sixteen-ounce sirloin. Nobody will know you're on a diet.

Just so you know, there's no law against ordering a nice piece of grilled fish at a steak house. You won't be blacklisted. Also watch out for the side dishes. You don't go to a steak house for the fries and creamed spinach; you're there for the meat. The sides are a necessary evil. Make sure some steamed asparagus hits the table in addition to everything else. And by that we don't mean swimming in

Urban Myth: *Weigh yourself every day.*

Urban Skinny: *Salt, hormones, getting off a plane, and, uh, how shall we say this, not taking a poop can make it look like you're failing, but you're not. Weigh yourself once a week at the same time, and assess your overall progress monthly so you don't get discouraged. Take measurements and know how your clothing fits. And check your body composition, because a pound of fat takes up more space than a pound of muscle.*

hollandaise, or a potato floating in sour cream and butter. All sauces can be ordered on the side. Avoid the dessert—it's just a business dinner. Skip the schlag! And if you know what that means, you know what we mean.

Sunday Brunch

Every urban dweller relishes the weekend brunch. Typically brunch occurs midday—sleep in, go late. Brunch is called brunch for a reason. It's not breakfast; it's not lunch. It's both. Combined. Which means you don't get brunch and then go home and eat lunch. The joy of brunch is that it's a nice time to indulge a little. Operative word being *little*. Don't go crazy. On a weekend, your typical day could be brunch, an afternoon snack, and dinner. So do the math; you can have half your calories for the day at brunch (approximately). And half doesn't mean all, it means half.

Pancakes and waffles come in wheat and whole-grain varieties these days. The calories are the same, but it's better to choose whole grain if possible; they are higher in fiber and will fill you up more than regular pancakes. Remember, fiber fills you up. Pick fresh berries over chocolate chips or the fruit compote. Berries are rich in antioxidants.

By now, all professional dieters have heard of the egg-white omelet, but you may actually be tired of it as your mainstay, and it's not always the lightest choice. Here's why: Sometimes it's slathered in oil to be cooked and loaded with more cheese than you need, and if you pick all the fillings, your omelet can add up. Egg whites themselves are great—just 20 calories each. But your egg-white omelet shouldn't be loaded up like a late-night drunken college pizza order. So if you want the egg-white omelet, load it with veggies, ask that it be cooked with spray, not oil, and ask for just a touch of cheese. Otherwise, here are some other options: eggs Benedict with the hollandaise on the side; if you just touch the tip of your fork into the sauce you'll get flavor in every bite. Eggs benny the Urban Skinny way is two poached eggs on the English muffin and a slice of Canadian bacon or fresh fruit. Canadian bacon is leaner than the regular kind—just half the calories. If you really need the real deal, a strip of bacon is only 50 calories. Just don't eat five pieces. Keep track and log what you eat.

Now those are some savory options. Sweet tooth hitting you? Ask your server for a short stack if you're craving pancakes. That means two versus three or four six-inch pancakes. A plain waffle is about 500 calories. Stuffed pancakes are stuffed with extra calories, so skip 'em. For both sweet choices, order the butter on the side or skip it altogether. And contrary to what you did when you were five years old, don't pour the syrup on your waffle or pancake until there is more syrup than waffle or pancake. Pour a little in a side bowl and dip, don't dunk.

> Antioxidants are substances found in certain foods like berries, tomatoes, and green tea. Since antioxidants zap the free radicals that may cause cancer, a diet rich in antioxidants may reduce your risk of developing certain types of cancer.

Guys' Night Out

Here's a special section for the Urban Skinny dude: Guys' night out isn't always the healthiest night of the week. Obviously, you're going to bond with your buddies, but let's have that game plan. Start with the drinks—opt for light beer instead of regular and save 50 calories a bottle. Doesn't sound like much, but be honest—are you out for a beer or five? Yes, we thought so. When it's your turn to buy a round, maybe grab a club soda with lime and nobody will know it's not a gin and tonic. And you're not a college kid anymore; pace yourself and drink slower than everyone else.

> A Bloody Mary or mimosa is about 150 calories (each, not both). Healthy bonus: Tomato products are rich in lycopenes, which may reduce the risk of developing certain cancers, including prostate. OJ contains antioxidants and has loads of vitamin C.

Okay, all-you-can-eat wing night sounds like a great idea, right? But did you know that one wing dipped in blue cheese has 100 calories? One. That's right. How many did you eat in college? Twenty?

Don't make the wings your dinner. Have a couple, then order the grilled chicken sandwich (not the bacon double cheeseburger). And skip the fries. Even if you're better behaved than all the guys at the table, a guys' night out might end up being a maintenance day, not a weight-loss day. We just don't want it to be a weight-gain day. Be cool and have fun.

Urban Recap

Be prepared ahead of time; if you get to pick the restaurant, pick whatever's easiest for you; and as you face various scenarios, use what you've learned to stay on track.

Up Next

You know how to order; now you need to know what to order whether you're eating Italian, Chinese, or French! An international passport to dining is the next step to being Urban Skinny.

CHAPTER 5

Tacos Are
Diet Food?

*Sarah, 39 years old, high-ranking finance executive, bicoastal—
LA/New York—spends more days eating in restaurants than not,
used to rarely drink water. One month last year, she slept in
hotels thirty out of thirty-one nights.*

Urban Challenge
*Sarah not only hits a lot of restaurants, she hits a lot of towns. A regular
month includes trips to seven or more different cities. She has offices
in two towns and often eats out—breakfast, lunch, and dinner. Control
over her food choices used to be a major obstacle, especially when hitting some of her ethnic faves.*

Urban Surprise
*Sarah knows she can actually lose weight. She lost 25 pounds once
when she tried the no-carb thing. Even though she got rid of a chunk of
weight, she put 40 pounds back on as soon as she started indulging in
bread and rice again. Sarah worked out, but not consistently.*

Urban Insight
*Exchanging the bagel for a slice of toast was just a part of Sarah's
success. She finally embraced ordering fish and sushi and learned
what different ethnic foods were smart choices, since not eating at*

restaurants all the time was simply not an option. She slimmed down by slimming her portions down, too. Sarah added a Luna bar as an afternoon snack instead of only eating lunch and feeling starved by dinner. She found an afternoon snack took the edge off and allowed her to make better choices when the menu was in front of her at 9:00 p.m. Since Sarah spent so much time on airplanes, she made a point of carrying her own food on board instead of being forced to eat what was dropped in front of her. She worked out more often and whenever possible she walked to work.

Smart Ethnic Choices

When you live in a major urban center, you have a hectic work life and busy social life. You probably eat out more than you eat in. And chances are that when you do eat in, you often wind up ordering takeout or delivery from the Chinese or Mexican place around the corner. Ordering can often pose a challenge when you're trying to shave off a few pounds, especially with ethnic cuisine. *Urban Skinny's* cuisine-by-cuisine guide will keep you on track. And yes, you can even eat Mexican food.

Here's the deal: Just because you're an aficionado of international cuisine doesn't mean you're allowed to treat every dinner out like you're on vacation. Little Italy doesn't require a passport, and Chinatown ain't checking your visa. So order like it's just another everyday meal.

The basic rules of "restauranting" we gave you in the previous chapters apply, but depending on which fare you choose, your order will vary. Let's embark on a trip around the world without leaving your neighborhood.

Mexican

The Urban Good

Most Mexican dishes are loaded with veggies—lettuce, tomato, and yes, even salsa count as vegetables. Guacamole is rich in heart-healthy oils, and beans are high in fiber. Americans consume an average of only 15 grams of fiber per day, but everyone should eat 25 to 35 grams daily. A cup of black beans gets you halfway there. But you still have to eat Mexican in moderation.

The Urban Bad

Mexican can be tricky for those trying to shed weight. It can be done, but you need to learn to navigate the menu so you don't eat more than your budgeted calories. More tempting than the bread basket you find in other restaurants are the guacamole, salsa, and chips that get dropped on most tables in a Mexican restaurant. It's part of the ritual and a tough one to pass on. And honestly, have you ever had just one chip? Once you start, it's hard to control yourself. The same can be said for the margaritas. One problem with Mexican food can be portion size. The entrées can vary from restaurant to restaurant, so you have to really look at them carefully. Besides, if you indulge in the chips, guac, and margs you might as well have just eaten half a loaf of bread before your meal (calorically speaking).

The Urban Ugly

In a Mexican restaurant, anything fried and topped with cheese will completely ruin your diet. Throw in the sour cream and it's uglier than ugly. The worst offenders include the chiles rellenos, enchiladas topped with a cream sauce, and queso with chorizo; you could be eating a day's-worth-of-calories entrée packed with sodium, cholesterol, and saturated fat. Otherwise known as a heart attack on a platter.

¿Tienes hambre?

URBAN INSIGHT: Throw the salsa on top of your salad and save some calories; it makes a decent salad dressing.

Taco Stand

Grilled fish taco: 150–170 calories (flour tortilla, fish, lettuce, tomato, salsa)
Chicken taco: 200 calories (flour tortilla, chicken, cheese, lettuce, tomato, salsa)
Beef taco: 200–250 calories (flour tortilla, beef, cheese, lettuce, tomato, salsa)

- ☐ Eat a corn tortilla instead of a flour one and save 50 calories.
- ☐ 4-inch flat tortillas are the standard, but don't forget to assess the size. Mexican can vary, so be honest with yourself when sizing up your plate.

Mixed green salad with non-creamy dressing on the side (2 tablespoons): 100 calories
Bowl tortilla soup: 200–250 calories
Flauta: 100–150 calories
Empanada: 200–300 calories
1 ounce tortilla chips: 150 calories (10–15 chips)
Traditional taco salad with shell: 1000+ calories
Quesadilla: 700–1500 calories total (small appetizer triangle, 3–4 knuckles wide at widest part, is 150 calories; ¼ of a quesadilla is 300 calories; as an entrée, eat half and request sour cream and guacamole on the side)

URBAN INSIGHT: Fish tacos are to West Coasters what dirty water dogs are to New Yorkers (sort of). If you want a fish taco, you can find one in the west. Luckily, tacos are a healthy pick for a quick bite. Fish, beef, or chicken tacos generally have two ounces of protein—and there's a little bit of everything, but only a pinch of the really bad-for-you things, like cheese. A taco could be a quick snack in the afternoon, or two could serve as a decent lunch.

Mexican Dinner

Best Appetizer Picks
Ceviche (2 ounces of fish, a few chunks of avocado): 150 calories
Mixed greens, with 2 tablespoons non-creamy dressing on the side: 100 calories

Bowl tortilla soup: 200—250 calories

Only If You're Sharing Appetizer Picks

¡Cuidado!

Flautas: 100–150 calories each

Fondido: Melted grease in a bowl can be *delicioso,* but it'll cost you 50 calories per dip.

Empanada: 200–300 calories

Guacamole (made with 2 avocados): 800 calories

Basket of 30 chips: 400–500 calories

> **A typical basket of tortilla chips has two to three ounces of chips, which can be as much as 450 calories.** Spice it up on the side: Salsa, pico de gallo, chile verde sauce: 0 calories
> Guacamole: 2 tablespoons equal 50 calories
> Sour cream: 2 tablespoons equal 60 calories

Best Entrée Picks

Grilled shrimp or fish: Always a good option, you will find this in most upscale Mexican places. Watch your sides, though: ½ cup of rice is 100 calories and so is ½ cup of beans. Watch your sauces, too; anything with cream can add more than 300 calories to your plate.

Fajitas, shrimp or chicken: 6–8 ounces protein have 250–300 calories, onion-and-pepper sauté 100 calories, each flour tortilla 100 calories. Some restaurants will allow you to order half beef and half chicken, so if you're craving beef, split the difference.

Taco salad: 4 ounces beef, chicken, or shrimp with lettuce, tomato, and cheese. Skip the shell and/or chips, and get your guacamole and sour cream on the side (dip lightly, don't dunk). That makes a traditional 1,000-calorie taco salad a nice 400–500 calorie modified one. And the nice thing about an old-fashioned taco salad is there's no dressing to mess with.

> **100-Calorie Add-Ons**
> 10 chips
> 5 chips dipped in guacamole
> ½ cup rice or black beans
> 1 shot of tequila
> 1 Corona Light
> 1 flour tortilla or 2 corn tortillas
> ¼ cup guacamole

URBAN INSIGHT: Most urban Mexican restaurants will give you crudités to dip with upon request—carrots in the guac instead of chips give you some crunch, satisfy your hunger, and save you mucho calories pre-dinner.

Gotta-Have-It Entrée Picks

Burrito: If you can't pick it up, and you need a fork and knife to eat it, it's likely more than 1,000 calories. Easy solutions: 1) Eat one-third to a half. 2) Skip the rice, since you're loading up on starch with the tortilla, and save 100 to 200 calories. 3) Eat just the inside if you can, because the tortilla alone has 300 calories. Add some veggies to the burrito to increase its girth, not your own. The key to ordering a burrito lies in modifying what they offer you on the menu.

Quesadilla: These can seriously vary from place to place. One triangle (measure 3–4 knuckles) of a quesadilla can run you about 150 calories. If this is your meal, eat half of an entire one (3–4 triangles), with all the extra junk on the side.

Urban Skinny 500-Calorie Quick Picks

Vegetable salad with 2 tablespoons non-creamy dressing, 2 soft fish tacos, 2 tablespoons guacamole, salsa

Vegetable salad with 2 tablespoons vinaigrette dressing, 4–6 ounces grilled fish or shrimp, steamed veggies and salsa, ½ cup of black beans

1 margarita on the rocks, salad with salsa as your dressing, 10–15 chips with ¼ cup guacamole

1 glass of sangria, 1 bowl tortilla soup, 5–10 chips and salsa

1 crunchy beef taco, 1 enchilada, salad with salsa

1 flauta, 1 empanada, 1 small triangle of quesadilla, salad with salsa

---

Drinks

Glass of sangria: 150–200 calories
Margarita on the rocks: 200 calories
Corona Light: 100 calories
Avoid frozen margaritas: 16 ounces equals 400 calories. Once you start adding the flavoring and sweetened syrups, you're looking at an additional 200 calories. So one big flavored frozen margarita can add up to 600 calories a drink, which for some of you is your entire dinner budget.

Try to stick to one low-cal drink with Mexican. If you must have two, make your second beverage a glass of wine or light beer. One margarita is the Urban Skinny way. Remember: If you have alcohol, you should skip the starch. Always order a margarita without salt on the rim—Mexican food is high in sodium already. If you weigh yourself the morning after a salty meal, you might see that you've retained anywhere from one to three pounds of water.

(Note: Those famous delicious Rosa Mexicana pomegranate margaritas are only 250 calories.)

Dessert

You don't go to a Mexican restaurant for dessert. Since it's not going to be the restaurant's specialty, you should probably skip it. Why waste a calorie on something that's average? If you ignore what you're reading right now, though, and order the flan or tres leches cake, have just one bite.

URBAN INSIGHT: If you have 10 average-sized chips and you truly dip, not dunk, them into the guacamole, you'll eat about $1/4$ cup of guacamole—about 250 calories altogether. If you dunk and really load your 10 chips up, you're eating more like 550 calories—an entire meal's worth of calories for many people.

Ordering-In Bonus

No guacamole and chips in your face, and nobody's mixing the house margaritas on demand. So if you really want Mexican food, but want to stay on track, have it delivered. *Olé!*

Japanese

The Urban Good

Japanese restaurants never have a bread basket on the table, they have crappy desserts (really, green tea ice cream?), sushi and sashimi have little to no added oil, fish and avocado are heart healthy, and many dishes use tons of veggies. Japanese food offers lots of low-calorie, high-volume picks; you can try a variety of little things and not bust your calorie budget (a bento box). They often serve limited cocktails, so you probably won't be tempted to over-drink (unless, of course, you're a fan of sake).

The Urban Bad

You gotta work hard to find "the bad" on a Japanese menu. Where you'll falter: quantity. Healthy doesn't mean all-you-can-eat, so be careful not to overeat. If you order sushi, it may seem easy to devour a few rolls, but that rice will expand in your stomach! Watch the fried foods like tempura, rock shrimp, and the spring rolls (when you see the word "crispy," take a cue—it's Japanese for fried).

The Urban Ugly

A diet high in sodium may increase your risk of developing high blood pressure (hypertension). Most sodium in your diet isn't coming from the salt-shaker, but from the processed food you're eating. "Low sodium" means less than 140 milligrams of sodium per serving.

Sodium is usually off the charts at a Japanese restaurant. You should limit intake to 2,300 milligrams of sodium a day (one teaspoon of salt). One tablespoon (a ½-ounce takeout package) of soy sauce has about 900 milligrams. Even the low-sodium version has 600 milligrams—lower, but by no means low. Watch your other sauces and dips, too. And since most of our sodium comes from the food we eat, not the salt we shake, take heed when it comes to Japanese. Miso soup, for example, has 500 milligrams of sodium. Seaweed comes from the sea; translation: salt water. You could easily salt yourself out with one meal.

Japanese Restaurant (or Takeout)

Sushi rolls and pieces can vary (if you have to use a fork and knife to cut your sushi, it's too big). Try to eyeball it and average out your pieces when you eat.

> The average American consumes 3,000–6,000 milligrams of sodium a day—that's up to double what they should take in.

Best Appetizer Picks

Seaweed salad typical serving: 100 calories
½ bowl of edamame (1 cup unshelled): 100 calories
Miso soup: 50 calories
Green salad with 2 tablespoons ginger dressing: 100 calories
Oshinki: 0 calories
Hijiki: 0 calories
Shumai (steamed veggie, shrimp, or wasabi): 35 calories each
Summer roll: 50 calories (100 with sauce)
Chicken satay: 50 calories per skewer

Only If You're Sharing Appetizer Picks

Rock shrimp: 20 calories each
Veggie tempura: 50–100 calories each
Fried dumpling: 100 calories each
Spring roll: 150 calories each

Best Entrée Picks (on average, based on one half ounce protein per piece)

Sashimi: 20–30 calories
Sushi (nigiri): 50 calories
Eel (anago) sushi: 80 calories
Tamago (egg): 70 calories
Fatty tuna sushi: 70 calories

Most pieces of sushi contain 1 tablespoon of rice, approximately 25–30 calories. The average sashimi piece is 20–30 calories (salmon has more calories than white fish); therefore the average piece of sushi (nigiri) with a half ounce of fish is about 50 calories.

Urban Skinny 500-Calorie Quick Picks

*Green salad with 2 tablespoons carrot ginger dressing
on the side
1 rainbow roll
1 piece of salmon sushi
1 piece of tuna sushi*

*Green salad with 2 tablespoons carrot ginger dressing
on the side
½ cup edamame shelled
1 tuna roll
3 pieces salmon sashimi*

*Miso soup
Salad with 2 tablespoons dressing on the side
½ cup edamame shelled
2 shrimp shumai
4 pieces of a roll or sushi (any) or 8 pieces sashimi*

*Salad with 2 tablespoons dressing on the side
Miso soup
1 piece eel sushi
1 shrimp tempura roll (6 pieces)*

Rolls

Rolls are usually made with ½ cup of rice per roll. There are big rolls and small. Most are cut into six pieces. Typically you can use the following numbers as a guideline:

Avocado roll: 150 calories (25 per piece)
Cucumber roll: 120 calories (20 per piece)
Tuna/cucumber roll (no rice): 120 calories (20 per piece)

California roll: 180–200 calories (about 30 per piece)

Tuna roll: 180 calories (about 30 per piece)

Spicy tuna roll: 250–300 calories (about 40–50 per piece)

Dragon roll: 250–300 calories (40–50 per piece)

Rainbow roll: 300-350 calories (50–60 per piece)

Shrimp tempura roll: 300 calories (50 per piece)

Salmon/avocado roll: 300 calories (about 50 per piece)

Eel/avocado roll: 360 calories (60 per piece)

Soy sauce, wasabi, and ginger add an insignificant number of calories.

> **100-Calorie Add-Ons**
> 2 pieces sushi
> 3–4 pieces sashimi
> ½ cup edamame shelled
> 1 piece eel sushi and 1 piece sashimi
> 3 steamed shumai
> Seaweed salad
> 2 summer rolls
> 2 chicken satay
> 1 fried dumpling
> 1–2 small pieces veggie tempura

Drinks

Sake (1 ounce): 40 calories

Sapporo (12 ounces): 140 calories

> **Sake option:** If you want 2 ounces (about 100 calories) of sake, order your roll without rice or stick to the sashimi.

Dessert

½ cup (1 scoop) green tea ice cream: 150–200 calories

½ cup red bean ice cream: 200–250 calories

1 mochi ball: 100 calories

Sorbet (½ cup or one scoop): 100 calories

Pineapple (¼ of a pineapple): 100–150 calories

You can always substitute brown for white rice to increase your fiber intake, but remember the calories remain the same.

Stick to the rules: Dip, don't dunk, into the soy sauce to keep sodium under control. And don't discourage yourself the next morning by jumping on the scale. Sushi = bloating.

**Attention pregnant women:
Go ahead and order your
sushi—most places will
cook the fish that others
are eating raw. Just ask!**

Ordering-In Bonus

There's no sake or Japanese beer. Remember that the fried stuff will be soggy by the time it gets to you, so don't even bother. You can't order that second or third roll just because you feel hungry.

Sushi Haters

If you hate sushi, but someone drags you to a sushi restaurant, keep in mind that chicken or shrimp teriyaki is about 200–300 calories and comes with steamed veggies. That bowl of rice on the side is about 300 calories, so eat accordingly.

Greek

The Urban Good

Greece doesn't have to mean grease! Greek food is jam-packed with plenty of whole grains, beans, and veggies, all of which are rich in fiber, vitamins, and minerals. It's high in heart-healthy oils, including olive oil, and there's usually a nice low-calorie grilled fish on a Greek menu.

The Urban Bad

Nearly every country has its cheese and Greece is no exception; feta should be eaten in moderation. Greek menus have a lot of beef and lamb options as well, which are higher in saturated fat, calories, and cholesterol than chicken or fish. And while Urban Skinny is a fan of the health benefits of olive oil, oil is also high in calories, so as with the meat and cheese, moderation and portion control are important. Watch your fish, too—it could be slathered in oil. Has anyone ever met a hummus and pita they didn't like? We thought not. Watch out—it's usually the first thing to land on your table.

The Urban Ugly

Dishes such as pastitsio and moussaka pack a big punch: Big portions of layered ground lamb, pasta, cheese, fried eggplant, and cream sauce! Pastitsio is often referred to as "Greek lasagna." It's not your friend.

URBAN INSIGHT: The medical world has long known the health benefits of a traditional Mediterranean diet, which typically consists of whole grains, plenty of veggies, and heart-healthy olives and olive oils.

Greek: In or Out

As with Mexican food, you can find "fast food" Greek food, as well as more upscale Greek restaurants in most cities.

100-Calorie Add-Ons
½ pita
2 grape leaves
1 ounce feta cheese
¼ cup hummus
10 large olives
¼ cup tzatziki
1 shot ouzo

Best Appetizer Picks

2-inch stuffed grape leaves (rice): 50–75 calories each

Greek salad (2 tablespoons feta and 2 tablespoons dressing): 200 calories

Grilled or marinated octopus (hot or cold): 200–250 calories

Grilled sardines: 200 calories

1 pita: 150–200 calories

2 tablespoons hummus: 50 calories

Olives: small 5 calories; large 10 calories each

1 tablespoon taramosalata: 60 calories

1 tablespoon tzatziki: 20 calories

Only If You're Sharing Appetizer Picks

Fried calamari: 500 calories per order

Greek spread platter (hummus, tzatziki, taramosalata, and 5–10 olives, ¼ cup each spread): 550 calories

Pita: 150–200 calories each

Spanakopita: 400 calories per order

Best Entrée Picks

(based on a 6-ounce portion)

Whole grilled or roasted white fish: 200–300 calories (*request little oil)

3 baby lamb chops: 350 calories

Roasted chicken without the skin (white meat only): 300–350 calories

Souvlaki or shish kebab: 250–300 calories (grilled and marinated lean chicken)

Lamb or beef kebab: 400–450 calories

Urban Skinny 500-Calorie Quick Picks
*Greek salad with 2 tablespoons feta, 1 grape leaf, 1
tablespoon dressing, 5 olives*
Simply grilled white fish, shrimp, or chicken kebab
Fresh steamed vegetables

Sharing the meze platter:
1 tablespoon each tzatziki, hummus, taramosalata, and ½ pita
Grilled or marinated octopus appetizer
Greek salad with 1 ounce feta, 3 olives, and no dressing

Vegetable salad with 1 tablespoon each feta and dressing
Half order moussaka
Side of steamed veggies

Gotta-Have-It Entrée Picks (but only eat half)

Gyro with lamb: 750–800 calories (including pita, but not sides like rice)
Moussaka: 800–1000 calories

URBAN INSIGHT: If you're dying for a glass of Boutari wine, pull the pita.

Italian

The Urban Good

Marinara sauce is rich in antioxidants, olive oil is heart healthy, and Italian dishes generally have lots of veggie options and salads. Even so, finding good in Italian (other than in the taste) is tough—moderation is key. You'll almost always find a fish option on an Italian menu.

The Urban Bad

Portion sizes are tough to battle, especially with the pasta; sauces can be heavy; and that bread basket is a tough one to pass up.

The Urban Ugly

Fried foods topped with Parmesan, such as chicken or eggplant, can really add up. Dishes with cheese and creamy sauces are not only high in calories, but also rich in artery-clogging oil.

Italian Dinner

Here's the bottom line on Italian: Unless you're ordering fish, it's all going to boil down to portion control. Less is more.

Best Appetizer Picks

Tricolor or arugula salad (add either a little shaved parm or olive oil on the side): 100–150 calories
Steamed artichoke (depends what you dip in): 100 calories
Minestrone soup (bowl): 200 calories
Melon with an ounce of prosciutto: 200 calories
Clams casino: 40 calories each

Only If You're Sharing Appetizer Picks

Fried calamari (5 rings): 100 calories (tentacles are double!)
Baked clams: 100–200 calories each, depending on size
Caesar salad appetizer: 300 for the entire thing
Mozzarella and tomato: 300–400 calories

Best Entrée Picks

6 ounces grilled fish or shrimp (usually served with steamed or grilled vegetables): 300–400 calories

Shrimp fra diavolo (spicy red sauce): 500 calories (eat all the seafood and pick at the pasta)

Zuppa di pesce: 500 calories (eat all the seafood and pick at the pasta)

100-Calorie Add-Ons
One slice crusty bread
1 golf ball–sized meatball
5 rings fried calamari
1 baked clam
Adding shaved Parmesan
1 cappuccino, biscotti
1 shot of sambuca
1 glass of Prosecco

Gotta-Have-It Entrée Picks

Something Parmesan: the entire order could take you for 1200 calories, not including the pasta on the side. You can take off about 200 calories if you opt for chicken instead of veal. So if you must have it, only consume one-third to half of an order. Make sure you ask for a side of spinach instead of the pasta that typically comes along with it.

Half order of pasta with Bolognese sauce: 400–500 calories

Large cheese ravioli with red sauce: 75 calories for a 2-inch-by-2-inch ravioli. Do the math once you see the order and ravioli size.

Pizza Options

Super thin crust pizza (Margherita brick-oven style): 100–150 calories for a slice (measure 3–4 knuckles wide)

Dessert

Cappuccino with low-fat milk: 50 calories

2 bite-size biscotti: 50 calories

Ricotta cheesecake: 500 calories (a true bite—50 calories)

Tiramisu: 500 calories (a true bite—50 calories)

Tartufo: 500 calories a bowl (try just a bite—don't dig for gold!)

Gelato is Italian for Häagen-Dazs: ½ cup or one scoop = 250–300 calories

Urban Skinny 500-Calorie Quick Picks
Tricolor salad with 2 tablespoons dressing on the side, grilled fish or shrimp, steamed broccoli rabe with a touch of Parmesan, one glass Chianti

Steamed artichoke (no dipping sauce), half order seafood risotto, veggie salad with 2 tablespoons non-creamy dressing on the side

Salad with aged balsamic, half order lasagna

Drinks

Shot grappa, sambuca, or limoncello with your espresso: 100 calories
Chianti: 150 calories per glass (4 glasses in a bottle)
Mangia!

URBAN INSIGHT: Make your dressing the aged balsamic—it's expensive for a reason and has no calories.

Ordering-In Bonus

The hot bread isn't calling your name, and it's easier to portion out a plate of pasta and put the rest in the fridge for the next day's lunch. There's no dessert tray walking by, either.

Steak House

The Urban Good

You can always order fish, and the preparation is usually simple, with fewer hidden ingredients, so measuring your calories is easier. Veggies aren't being rationed, and a plain baked potato is not just an option but a delicacy. You can make requests for cooking style.

The Urban Bad

Red meat is high in calories and saturated fat, and it can be hard to resist when you keep smelling other people's entrées as they leave the kitchen. Watch the creamy side dishes.

The Urban Ugly

A fifty-two-ounce porterhouse. Need we say more? Two people usually eat a steak that could feed four. Sauces like béarnaise or Roquefort will only add to your diet misery.

Steak Dinner

What you see is likely what you get at a steak house. Basic dishes are usually grilled, simple, and sauceless. Green salads are at your finger-tips. Eyeball your protein portions.

Best Appetizer Picks

House salad or tomato and onion with 2 tablespoons non-creamy dressing on the side: 100 calories
Shrimp cocktail: 150–200 calories
Lump crab: 100–150 calories

> Cocktail or seafood sauce is low in calories and rich in lycopenes (antioxidants), which may reduce the risk of prostate cancer. It's high in sodium, though, so don't drink the stuff.

Only If You're Sharing Appetizer Picks

Seafood tower: clams, a bite of lobster, crab claw, and one shrimp—approximately 25 calories each (watch your side dips and stick to a squeeze of lemon and a dip of cocktail sauce)
Thick-cut slice of bacon (2 ounces): 200 calories

Best Entrée Picks

Grilled white fish is always the best: 200–300 calories for a 6-ounce serving. The same portion of salmon is more like 300–400 calories. Heads up: Places like the Palm might still hit you with large portions. You may have ordered fish, but you're not out of the water yet—sometimes the serving can be as big as a pound.

A 16-ounce New York strip (sirloin) shrinks to 12 ounces cooked (that's what will be sitting on your plate): Cut it in half and it's 350 calories. How happy will Fido be?

Petite filet: 8 ounces uncooked, 6 ounces cooked, 450 calories.

URBAN INSIGHT: **At a steak house, they usually tell you up front on the menu how big a piece of meat you're ordering. Remember that this number includes the bone and fat, before the piece is cooked. Once it's cooked, protein shrinks 25 percent. Eight ounces on the menu will be six ounces on the plate.**

Be nice to your arteries by consuming red meat in moderation. It's not only high in calories, but saturated fat and cholesterol, too.

Gotta-Have-It Entrée Picks

Filet mignon (16 ounces): 900 calories, if you eat the entire thing

Porterhouse (24-ounce porterhouse shrunk from cooking and minus 4 ounces of bone): 1100 calories

What did you learn about steak? You don't need to eat everything in front of you if you're trying to lose weight. And don't forget to trim all visible fat.

URBAN INSIGHT: **Watch it—some places put butter on the beef or offer you sauces like béarnaise or au poivre, which can add anywhere from 100 to 400 calories to your cut of beef. Remember, you're not going to a steak house for the sauce. Dijon mustard is a great alternative for dipping; there's nothing to it. Steak sauce won't add up too quickly either. They're both low-calorie options as long as you don't drown your meat.**

Urban Skinny 500-Calorie Quick Picks

Salad with 2 tablespoons non-creamy dressing on the side, 6 ounces swordfish, half a baked potato with a pat of butter, steamed asparagus

Half a 16-ounce sirloin (uncooked weight), steamed asparagus, and a glass of wine

Tomato onion salad with dressing on the side, petite filet, and steamed asparagus.

Good Sides

Baked potato: 200–300 calories
Dollop of sour cream: 100 calories
Pat of butter: 50–100 calories
Steamed asparagus (skip the hollandaise): 0 calories

Not-So-Good Sides—Make Sure You're Sharing!

Creamed spinach (just one spoonful plopped on your plate): 150 calories
French fries (20 fries, about 1 cup): 300 calories
Garlic mashed potatoes (½ cup): 150 calories
(Quick measure: Usually a spoonful of any side can be rounded off to 150 calories.)

100-Calorie Add-Ons

3–4 ounces lobster tail (surf and turf, anyone?)
3–4 jumbo shrimp
10 skinny fries, 5 steak fries
1 dinner roll
1–2 tablespoons béarnaise sauce
½ cup sautéed onions or mushrooms

Drinks

Light beer: 100 calories
Scotch on the rocks: 200 calories
Martini: 200 calories
Cabernet: 150 calories per glass
Gin or vodka and soda (not tonic): 100 calories

Dessert

Slice of chocolate cake: 500–600 calories
New York cheesecake: 500+ calories

Ordering-In Bonus

If you want beef and you're getting takeout, grab a burger. Skip the fries and you're looking at 600 calories.

Chinese

The Urban Good

Chinese food menus have no shortage of veggies, and butter and cream are not traditional to Chinese cooking. You do have to watch the grease factor when you order, though, because other oils are used. You can opt for brown rice, which is a good source of fiber, instead of white. There's not much on your menu in terms of dessert and a fortune cookie has just 30 calories.

The Urban Bad

Some Chinese dishes are deep-fried and most are high in sodium because of the soy and hoisin sauces. Soups are loaded with sodium too. Since there's a lot of sharing, the portions, like the nation, are humongous. Even if a dish is simply white-meat chicken sautéed with veggies, oil, and hoisin sauce, the serving size is usually too large for one person. Translation: too many calories to eat the entire order.

The Urban Ugly

Three words of evil: General Tso's chicken. One order weighs in at a whopping 1600 calories! If you must have it, ask that it be made with all white meat and sautéed instead of fried, and you'll whittle the order down to 800 calories. Call a friend because you still need to share it. Also, some restaurants fry in trans fats.

Chinese Food

Not always, but most often, Chinese is a takeout or delivery order. The upside of takeout is you can scoop a reasonable portion onto a plate and put the rest in the fridge for tomorrow's lunch. You won't be sitting at a table with a giant container of moo shu in front of you screaming, "Eat more!"

Best Appetizer Picks

1 cup hot-and-sour soup: 100–150 calories (low in calories but high in sodium; skip the fried noodles—one small bag is about 200 calories and 15 grams of fat)
Steamed vegetable dumplings: 50–100 calories each

Only If You're Sharing Appetizer Picks

Fried dumplings: 100–150 calories each

Peking duck (1 pancake with ¼ cup duck): 250 calories

Egg roll: 350 calories (cut it in half and save 175 calories, or better yet, cut it open and just eat the inside stuff)

Best Entrée Picks

(most containers from Chinese takeout hold 2–3 cups*)

Moo shu chicken or shrimp: 200–250 calories per cup

Chicken/shrimp and veggies sautéed with sauce: 250 calories per cup

Chicken chow mein: 200 calories per cup

Steamed chicken/shrimp with veggies: 200 calories for entire order, plus an additional 100 calories per ¼ cup sauce on the side; quickly toss the dish with the sauce and serve—you'll never miss the extra sauce

* Container sizes vary, so take the time to measure your food and then dump it on the plate. Don't stand at the counter and eat out of the container.

100-Calorie Add-Ons

1 triangle of scallion pancake

1 fried spring roll

½ cup rice

1 large steamed veggie dumpling

2 small veggie dumplings

1 cup egg-drop soup

1 cup wonton soup, 2 wontons

Urban Skinny 500-Calorie Quick Picks

1 order steamed chicken/shrimp with ¼ cup sauce (any)
1 cup brown rice or 2 large steamed veggie dumplings

1 cup hot-and-sour soup
Half order moo shu chicken
1 pancake and 1 tablespoon hoisin

1 cup hot-and-sour soup
Half order chicken and mixed veggies in brown or garlic sauce

---

Gotta Have It Entrée Picks

Orange beef: 400–500 calories per cup

Lemon chicken: 300–400 calories per cup

Cold sesame noodles: 400–500 calories per cup

French

The Urban Good

French restaurants often have tasting menus so you can have a few small bites of several delish things. Small portions are the norm. Many French menus have seafood options that keep calories in check.

The Urban Bad

"Fromage" means cheese, which means high calories. French cuisine also offers many artery-clogging options like roast duck, which has 25–30 grams of fat and 1500 calories. Sauces like béchamel, velouté, hollandaise, beurre blanc, mornay, béarnaise, and espagnole sound delectable, but you don't need a French–English dictionary to translate: Most are made from a roux base, which is—how shall we say it—flour and fat.

> If you're on a 1500-calorie-a-day diet, you should consume between 40 and 50 grams of fat a day (not a meal!).

You may sound oh so continental when you order au beurre (with butter), au gratin (with cheese), en croûte (wrapped in pastry), or graisse (fat or greased), but do so only if you want to be the size of France. Quiche is not a light lunch. A slice (500–800 calories) can be as hard on your calorie budget as buying euros is to your vacation budget.

Most people love cheese so much they want to marry it. Try to skip the cheese course after a rich French dinner. Cheese contains 100 calories per one-inch cube. Most cheese courses offer a minimum of three cheeses, each weighing at least an ounce. Some cheese courses will contain more calories than your entire fish entrée. If you absolutely need a piece of chèvre, order it—simply take a sliver, skip the bread, and call it dessert.

The Urban Ugly

You wanna watch the steak frites, steak au poivre, and steak with béarnaise. Beef is a tough enough pick when you're trying to lose weight, but dump some rich and creamy sauce on top and you

> Request steamed or grilled veggies, or ratatouille to complement your fish or chicken.

could be eating your entire day's worth of calories in one meal—just in your beef, the sides are extra. You're looking at taking in 1000 calories and between 30 and 40 grams of fat. Oh, and about the foie gras: Fat doesn't even begin to describe this one.

French Food: Parlez-Vous Petite?

The main difference between the way the French eat and the way Americans eat comes down to portions. French food is rich and great tasting. We say they eat small portions. What they really eat are proper portions. Take a tip from the French—think petite. Don't eat French food American style. (Less is more.)

Best Appetizer Picks

Simple salad or artichoke vinaigrette with 2 tablespoons dressing on the side: 100 calories

Moules (steamed mussels) small order: 150–200 calories if you skip the bread dipping!

Fish tartare: 100–150 calories

Half dozen oysters on the half shell: 120–150 calories

Bouillabaisse (fish soup): 150 calories per cup

Onion soup without the gratin (sprinkle a little Parmesan cheese): 400 calories with cheese, 200 calories without

100-Calorie Add-Ons
1 piece of French bread
4-ounce glass of wine
10 mussels (moules)
10 skinny fries
1–2 tablespoons of your favorite sauce
1 ounce cheese
2–3 thin slices saucisson

Only If You're Sharing Appetizer Picks

Frisée salad with lardons, croutons, and eggs, simply enjoy sans the dressing: 250 calories

Foie gras: 130 calories for 2 tablespoons (although it's served for one, it's best to share with at least one other person; think butter, not cream cheese, and just take a dab)

Urban Skinny 500-Calorie Quick Picks

Simple salad (2 tablespoons non-creamy dressing)
Grilled or poached white fish
Steamed veggies
1 glass of Chablis or Bordeaux

Chicken paillard (dressing on the side)
1 glass of Chablis or Bordeaux

Tuna tartare
Capon (no skin)
Steamed veggies

Appetizer portion of moules
10 fries (small handful)
Salad with 2 tablespoons of dressing

French onion soup
Salad with 2 tablespoons of dressing

Pommes frites sound fancy, but they contain the same calories as the McDonald's version: ½ cup adds up 230 calories

Fondue (dip, don't dunk, and stick with crudités and limit your bread and the meat dips): 25 calories per dip with veggies, 50 calories with bread or meat

Escargot: 30–50 calories each, and don't forget to shake (the butter, we mean) — if you sop up all the butter with bread, you've just eaten 500 more calories

"En papillote" means steamed in paper, always a good choice; poached, au jus, and aux herbes are also good choices.

Best Entrée Picks

(based on 6 ounces of protein)

Say *adieu* to full orders. Skip all those nasty sauces, or at the very least order them on the side and do a rather dainty fork dip into them every other bite. Better yet, with most French dishes you can share with *un ami* (a friend!) to create those tiny French portions found mostly in France.

Tuna niçoise (2 hard-boiled eggs, 4 ounces tuna, potatoes, a few olives, dressing on the side): 400 calories before dressing

Dover sole, halibut, or trout: 200–300 calories

Salmon: 300–400 calories

Roasted chicken (remove skin): 200 calories; eat just the breast

Pot-au-feu (stewed chicken) or coq-au-vin (chicken in wine), ask for white meat and remove the skin: 400 calories

Gotta Have It Entrée Picks

1 cup cassoulet: 500 calories

Steak frites (all the steak, half the fries): 600 calories

Duck à l'orange (size of deck of cards, with skin): 350 calories

Thai

The Urban Good

Loaded with vegetables, fairly low in calories, and rich in fiber. Many dishes are made with lean sources of protein like chicken, seafood, and shellfish. Traditional Thai spices give the food a flavor boost without a calorie boost. Thai is one of those cuisines you can share with friends so you can keep your portion size down and still try a bunch of things without overeating.

The Urban Bad

Watch the apps—there are lots of fried options, and if they're fried in trans fats, which they may very well be, you risk a rise in your cholesterol.

> **Trans fats (hydrogenated vegetable oils) are the worst of all the fats. They increase your bad cholesterol levels (LDL) and decrease the protective or good cholesterol levels (HDL).**

The Urban Ugly

Coconut milk is a big Thai ingredient—even in soups and most of the curries. Coconut is one of only two plant sources of saturated fat, which can increase your LDL levels (the bad cholesterol) the same way things like meat, bacon, and whole milk products do. Raw coconut milk packs a whopping 500 calories and 50 grams of artery-clogging fat per eight fluid ounces—ouch! Make sure you ask about ingredients before you order and try to get something without it.

Thai Food

Thai is sharable, so you can taste lots of good things but stick with small portions. There are many high-protein options and many times serving sizes aren't outrageous. As with other ethnic foods, though, be wary, as portion sizes and oil levels vary from place to place—not all pad thai is created equal.

Many Thai dishes use a curry sauce. Curry is a spice, so in and of itself, it doesn't contain any calories. The problem is that most curry dishes contain coconut milk, which adds a ton of calories and fat. Here's the solution: Serve yourself the chicken or shrimp with veggies with a slotted spoon or a fork. The coconut broth is very thin, and since the chicken or shrimp isn't breaded, most of the sauce ends up back in the dish—which is fine; it's not supposed to be soup! A typical dish has 6 ounces of lean protein, which is 200–250 calories. Here's the scoop on sauces:

- Green or red curry with chicken/seafood (6 ounces protein with minimal sauce): 300–350 calories

- Green or red curry with pork/beef (6 ounces protein with minimal sauce): 500–600 calories

- Massaman chicken curry (6 ounces protein with minimal sauce): 400–450 calories (a little more since it also has potato)

100-Calorie Add-Ons

½ cup jasmine rice
2 chicken satay skewers
2 steamed veggie dumplings
2 cups tom yum soup
2 tablespoons peanut sauce
2 small veggie or shrimp
    summer rolls
1 steamed meat dumpling
1 fried veggie dumpling
1 cup lemongrass soup
1 chicken lettuce wrap
    (3 tablespoons filling)
1 fried spring roll

Best Appetizer Picks

Chicken satay (3 ounces): 150 calories (it's usually already made with a little peanut sauce on it, so no need for extra dipping; 1 tablespoon peanut sauce contains 50–70 calories)

Vegetable or shrimp summer rolls (finger length): only 50–75 calories each

Steamed veggie dumplings: 50 calories each

Steamed meat dumplings: 75 calories each

Tom yum soup (clear broth soup with veggies): 50 calories per cup

Lemongrass soup: 100 calories per cup

Vegetable salad with 2 tablespoons peanut dressing on the side: 150 calories

Papaya salad with 2 tablespoons lime dressing on the side: 150 calories

Chicken lettuce wrap: 75–100 calories

Only If You're Sharing Appetizer Picks

Fried veggie dumplings: 75–100 calories each

Fried chicken/pork dumpling: 100–150 calories each

Fried spring roll: 100–150 calories each

Best Entrée Picks

Typically entrée containers hold about 2–3 cups; sometimes Thai servings are smaller than Chinese ones.
Thai basil chicken: 200–250 calories per cup
Thai basil beef: 250–300 calories per cup
Lemongrass chicken: 200–250 calories per cup
Spicy Thai beef salad (based on 4-ounce lean sirloin and 4 tablespoons dressing on the side): 500 calories

Gotta-Have-It Entrée Picks

Noodle/rice orders are usually 2–3 cups—remember ½ cup of either plain is 100 calories.
Pad see ew (noodles with fish sauce and thick soy sauce with chicken): 350 calories per cup
Pad thai (noodles pan-fried with egg, peanuts, and either chicken, tofu, or seafood): 400 calories per cup
Khao pad (Thai fried rice with shrimp, seafood, pork, crab, and beef): 350 calories per cup

Thai on the Side

Jasmine rice: 200 calories per cup
Sticky rice: 250–300 calories per cup (be mindful: some sticky rice is made with coconut milk, which will double the calorie content)
Cucumber salad with 2 tablespoons dressing on the side: 100 calories per cup

---

Urban Skinny 500-Calorie Quick Picks
Pad thai, 1 cup
Veggie salad with 2 tablespoons dressing

1 order chicken curry (scoop the meat, leave the sauce behind)
1 cup jasmine rice

1 order chicken satay
1 cup lemongrass soup
2 chicken lettuce wraps

Indian

The Urban Good

One of India's cooking techniques, the tandoor, is great for low-fat cooking. No extra oil is used and still the food comes out moist and flavorful. Lean protein choices are all over Indian menus, and the spiciness of the food might in fact prompt you to eat less than you would with blander foods.

The Urban Bad

The spice is double-edged: You might eat less, but when you want to cut the heat from what you have eaten, you'll turn to bread—and on an Indian menu, the choices are endless. Nan bread, poori, paratha—and then there's the rice. So remember your servings when partaking. You'll see some fried foods on the menu as well—deep-fried in fact. Samosas, pakoras, and papadum are yummy, but seriously caloric.

The Urban Ugly

Some of the main ingredients in Indian food, like cream and coconut milk, can really slam your calorie count. Watch out for menu picks like malai, muglai, korma, tikka masala, and saag paneer. Even if you're ordering vegetarian dishes, you're not necessarily ordering low-calorie dishes. The words aren't interchangeable, especially with Indian food. Paneer—cheese—adds an extra punch. Be aware.

Indian Food

Some places will honor your request to have your food prepared without oil and will even use yogurt in place of cream. But be a detective here—if it tastes like oil, it is. Watch the nan bread—it can come slathered in cheese, oil, and other treats, so even a small piece can mess up your math.

Best Appetizer Picks

Chicken or fish tikka: 150 calories
Shrimp balchao (pickled): 100–150 calories if you just eat 3 large shrimp and ease up on the tomato sauce

Hot pickles: 150 calories per ½ cup

Bowl vegetable soup: 100–150 calories

Chutney: 75–100 calories per 2 tablespoons

Bowl mulligatawny soup (ask first if there's cream): 200 calories without cream, double with cream

Bhindi bhajee (okra in tomato sauce): 100 calories per cup

> **100-Calorie Add-Ons**
> 2–3 tablespoons of chutney
> ½ cup rice
> ½ cup dhal
> 1 pakora
> 1 chapati

Only If You're Sharing Appetizer Picks

Samosa: 150 calories for a small one, 250 for a large one

Dhal: 120 calories per ½ cup

Papadum: 55 calories for 4 inches in diameter

Pakora: 100–150 calories each

Best Entrée Picks

Tandoor anything is great—chicken, white fish, or shrimp tandoori: 200–300 calories depending on size

Fish spiced (ask for no coconut milk): 250–300 calories

White-meat chicken vindaloo (spicy!): 400 calories for 6 ounces (dark meat about 150 calories more)

White-meat chicken tikka or kebabs: 250–350 calories

Half order of lamb or beef tandoori: 250–300 calories

> ## Urban Skinny 500-Calorie Quick Picks
> *Mixed greens with 2 tablespoons of non-creamy dressing*
> *Chicken tandoor*
> *1 small triangle nan*
>
> *Half portion of chicken tikka masala (skip the sauce and just pluck out the meat)*
> *½ cup rice*
>
> *1 small samosa*
> *Chicken tikka kebab*

Gotta Have It Entrée Picks

Saag (palak) paneer: 150–200 calories per ½ cup, but a typical order of this dish of cheese with spinach and cream can pack in 800 calories
Biryanis: 250–300 calories per cup
Chicken tikka masala (it's the sauce that will add up here): 350–400 calories for a few ounces of chicken plucked out of the sauce

Indian Sides

Basmati rice: 200 calories per cup
Tamarind: 200 calories per cup
Nan: 150 calories for 1 triangle plain, baked in the tandoor
Paratha (buttered and layered bread): 200–250 calories for 1 triangle (stuffed with potato, meat, or cheese is upwards of 300–350 calories per triangle)
Whole-wheat poori (deep fried): 110 calories for 4 inches in diameter (size varies, so be aware)
Chapati (requested without butter): 100–125 calories for a medium slice; this is the lightest of bread choices
Raita (yogurt sauce): 60 calories for ½ cup

Urban Recap

Choose smart, order smart, and be honest when sizing up a portion. Restaurant sizes can vary—portions can be huge—so keep in mind that three ounces of protein measures up to a deck of cards. Watch the sauces and the sides everywhere; they can add up. When in doubt, you can't go wrong asking for grilled seafood or chicken and some veggies.

Up Next

Keeping your home in order from a food standpoint is as important as keeping on top of all your other household chores. Even though you're a rock star and don't have to spend too many nights at home, you might have to be there on occasion. There's an Urban Skinny method to keeping your kitchen stocked to help you avoid any food madness.

CHAPTER 6

So, Cooking's Not
Your Strong Suit . . .

Shelly, age 32, not super tall, event planner

Urban Challenge

Shelly works for a hip national magazine, which means she has to entertain clients with dinner and booze anywhere from two to four nights a week. The clients aren't the only ones who are hitting the liquor; pre–Urban Skinny, Shelly was a 20-drink-a-week girl. She also has to fly to Chicago or LA a couple of times a month without a lot of notice, which always ruined her exercise routine. To make matters worse, her kitchen held nothing substantial to eat—she didn't shop because she didn't know when she'd be around. When she was home she ate crap because she hadn't prepared to eat right.

Shelly's dad died when she was in her twenties, around the same time she moved to New York and started a high-stress job. On top of that, Shelly was a chubby kid and still suffers from what experts call "fat kid" syndrome. Since she'd tried so many diets, she was really hesitant to begin Urban Skinny. She was convinced she'd fail, an attitude that researchers feel is one of the major reasons people don't succeed.

Urban Surprise

The only way Shelly could lose weight was to completely retreat from her life. She'd lock herself inside her apartment and focus on one thing—following another fad diet. Each time, she'd come out 20 pounds lighter because of her micro-focus. But once she jumped back in and resumed her life, she couldn't keep it off. She'd always gain it back and then some. At one point, she even turned to diet drugs to help her get ahead.

Urban Insight

Shelly knocked off 15 pounds in a few months and was surprised that she was still able to stick to her social schedule. She cut the alcohol intake, and seven months after she began, she was down almost 28 pounds. She kept helpful food stocked at home so she didn't get screwed up when she came home to an empty fridge. A couple of months later, she popped up slightly but quickly got herself back on track by noticing that she had eased back into the drinking and that had cost her some pounds.

Shelly not only dropped three clothing sizes, she lowered her cholesterol as well. After she spent five months flat—not gaining, but not losing—Shelly kicked the exercise into high gear, making sure she did five hours a week of cardio, up from three and a half. She also really focused in on portion sizes and broke free of her plateau. Almost two years to the day after Shelly began, she was holding strong 37 pounds lighter. It'll be slow and steady, but Shelly plans to knock off a dozen more.

The Urban Skinny Kitchen

It's not often someone as fabulous as you stays home, but once in a while you find you need a break from your hectic social life. If it's raining, you don't want to ruin your new Jimmy Choo's by stepping in a puddle, so why leave the shelter of your living room? If there's a *Project Runway* marathon on Bravo, why get off the couch when the thought of a dozen back-to-back episodes makes you giddy?

Sometimes you don't choose to stay home, but circumstances force you in, like when dinner plans fall through at the last minute. Or you're expecting last week's date to call, so you leave your calendar wide open in case he wants to take you somewhere painfully trendy to tell you he's majorly into you (he'll call tomorrow—don't worry!).

When circumstances keep you home, you need to be food-ready so that you don't fall off the Urban Skinny wagon. And city dwellers, especially New Yorkers, know there are dangerous distractions morning, noon, or midnight with the world of delivery just a dial away. A bagel and cream cheese and a coffee can be delivered to your door faster than you can hit the toaster button. A burger and fries is just ten digits away. Chinese food is on your speed dial. And we're guessing when you say you "cooked" last night, you mean you scrambled an egg. How about that bachelorette concoction you call dinner? Boiling a handful of pasta and dumping a can of soup on it? Admit it—you've done it.

Urban Skinny knows that you have to be prepared for these situations. Don't come home after a twelve-hour workday and eat just cereal because it's the only thing on hand. You want to eat something balanced and satisfying. Change your habits, and get the closet you call your kitchen in order. We know you're busy, so we're not asking you to become Bree from *Desperate Housewives.* We're just saying to give yourself a fighting chance when you walk in the door.

Every Urban Skinny kitchen should include the basics:

- ☐ peanut butter (creamy or crunchy)—any kind you like— Skippy, Jif, or fresh is fine, or any other nut butter
- ☐ nonstick cooking spray
- ☐ olive oil and canola oil, or even sesame oil, for some extra flavor in your stir-fry
- ☐ 100% whole-wheat English muffins
- ☐ almonds, slivered or whole
- ☐ oatmeal packets or express bowls
- ☐ eggs

- ☐ individual cheese slices (not the processed kind)—you can get Swiss or any kind you like deli sliced

- ☐ string cheese or other 1-ounce individually packaged cheese

> Cereal with more than 4 grams of fiber per serving is a good pick. Fiber fills you up and keeps you regular.

- ☐ yogurt (low-fat or nonfat)—good brands: Stonyfield Farm, Horizon, Fage Total, Chobani

- ☐ Kashi (individual cups or a box) or other high-fiber cereals

- ☐ frozen waffles: Van's, Kashi Go Lean

- ☐ individually sized Bear Naked granola

- ☐ Hellmann's canola or light mayo

- ☐ your favorite non-creamy salad dressing (always on the side and measured)

- ☐ all-fruit jam

- ☐ skim milk

- ☐ frozen meals, such as Amy's, Lean Cuisine, Weight Watchers Smart Ones, FreshDirect Heat & Eat, Healthy Choice, or any frozen entrées that fit within your calorie budget and are healthy choices for meals—read the label

- ☐ favorite fresh veggies

- ☐ fresh fruit: stock up on your faves

- ☐ nitrate-free sliced deli meats

- ☐ frozen veggie burgers, tofu nuggets: Boca, Morningstar Farms, Amy's

> Nitrates in foods (preservatives) may increase your risk of developing certain types of cancer.

- ☐ canned soup (reduced or low sodium)

- ☐ edamame

- ☐ salsa

- ☐ hummus—pre-packaged single serving sizes are best (if not, scoop a measured serving into a little dish, pull out the crudités, step away from the hummus container, and sit down and eat)
- ☐ cottage cheese: 0 or 1% milk fat
- ☐ whipped butter (creates an illusion since it looks the same as non-whipped but has 30–40 fewer calories per tablespoon)
- ☐ protein powder, if you're a smoothie groupie
- ☐ tuna—bags are pre-measured, no draining needed
- ☐ individually packed pre-made brown rice (you pay a premium for convenience, but you'll save in the long run when you don't have to spend $200 buying a new pair of fat jeans)
- ☐ bars—Balance, ZonePerfect, Greens+, Luna, Lärabar, Nature Valley Sweet & Salty
- ☐ mini packets of raisins
- ☐ pickles
- ☐ Chef Paul Prudhomme's Blackened Redfish Magic blackening spices

URBAN INSIGHT: If you're not home very much, don't fill the fridge with a lot of berries, but pick fruits that last longer. Apples, grapes, and oranges can sit in the fridge for ten days and be fine. Berries will start to rot in just a couple of days.

Notice that chips, cookies, cupcakes, and ice cream aren't on the list. That's because you won't eat them if they're not there. Don't defeat yourself early by lining your kitchen with unlimited temptations.

Now, Urban Skinny is pretty clear—you can in fact eat just about anything you want to as long as you spread your calories properly throughout the day, you focus on portion control, and you don't over-spend your food budget. But by having some easy "go-to's" at home, you give yourself an extra chance to stay on track. Losing weight is not easy, so why make it even harder by forcing yourself to come home and stare down that gigantic container of ice cream? Don't create a battle for yourself. If you're hungry, you'll eat what's in front of you just because it is there, so give yourself a fighting chance by having the right tools at your fingertips.

URBAN INSIGHT: If you need snacks in your house, the 100-calorie prepackaged ones are great to get your sweet fix and keep your portion in check. And, uh, you eat only one—not ten or the entire box!

Whatever your treat is—pudding pops, sugar-free or fat-free Jell-O, or low-calorie ice-cream sandwiches—you get to buy one package at a time. When it's empty (which should happen over the course of a week, not a night), you can go buy another box of something. The only thing you should be buying in bulk is toilet paper and paper towels. The more junk you have in your house, the more you'll eat.

URBAN INSIGHT: If you have a grocery delivery service like FreshDirect or Peapod, you can avoid the impulse buys at the grocery store by ordering everything online. You can't grab for that giant bag of Kettle corn at the register when you fill your cart online. Never shop hungry—virtually or in person.

Also keep in mind that the following count as cooking:

- ☐ Scramble two eggs, add some salsa, Frank's RedHot sauce, and 1 ounce of cheese, and throw it in a whole-wheat pita. We city folk call that dinner. 500 calories.
- ☐ Take a Purdue low-fat breaded cutlet (1 cutlet is 120 calories) and toss it in the oven. Slice it up, throw it on a salad, or make some chicken parm by adding a couple of spoonfuls of your favorite tomato sauce (30 calories) and 2 tablespoons of shredded mozzarella cheese (50 calories). You'll have an Italian feast without the pan to clean and a 200-calorie serving. Add one cup of cooked pasta and a side of steamed veggies for a solid meal.

Economical, At-Home Quickie Dinners

400- to 500-Calorie Quickie Dinners (pick one from each column)

Urban Skinny Version	Protein (protein is measured cooked)	Fat	Starch	Veggies
Burger	4–6 ounces ground turkey breast 4 ounces chicken Veggie burger 4 ounces lean beef	1 ounce cheese ¼ avocado	whole-wheat English muffin roll	sprouts pickles tomato mushroom onions salsa
Omelet	2 eggs 6 egg whites 8 ounces liquid egg substitute	1 ounce cheese	2 slices whole-wheat dry toast	veggies
Stuffed potato (sweet or plain) medium size	4 ounces turkey 4 ounces diced chicken ½ cup chili ¾ cup cottage cheese Londoners—tuna and sweet corn topping without the mayo 3 ounces sirloin	1½ ounces cheese		steamed spinach mushrooms broccoli
Salad	6 ounces tuna 6 ounces chicken 7 ounces tofu	2 ounces vinaigrette or 2 tablespoons nuts and 1 ounce vinaigrette	½ cup chickpeas/beans or ½ cup corn	lettuce and other favorites for salad
Stir-fry	6 ounces chicken 4 ounces lean beef 4 ounces lean pork 6 ounces shrimp	1 tablespoon oil	1 cup brown rice	mushrooms zucchini onions

Add a side of steamed veggies to any of these dishes

□ In a bowl toss ¼ to ½ pound of fresh or frozen shrimp with a tablespoon of oil and some blackening spice. Heat a pan, add the shrimp, and cook until pink. Make a nice colorful side salad and pour a glass of Pinot Grigio, and you have a seven-minute dinner with less than 500 calories.

□ Heat up Amy's pre-made chili (300 calories' worth) if you don't have your own favorite recipe. Top it with ¼ cup of shredded cheddar and a dollop of nonfat sour cream. Sprinkle some diced onions or scallions on top, throw in some lettuce, and you just made a taco salad.

□ Craving pasta? If you need a pasta fix, don't make it from scratch—portion control will be too difficult. Instead, hit the pre-packaged, frozen, calorie-counted version. If you like to cook and you can use pasta power portion control, make yourself a cup and a half cooked noodles and top it with one cup of a red (tomato-based) lean turkey meat–based sauce.

Urban Myth: *Cooking at home means you have to have a ton of ingredients; it must be gourmet and you must follow a recipe from a famous chef's book.*

Urban Skinny: *This counts as cooking: Go to your favorite gourmet grocery and grab a pre-cooked piece of salmon, tuna, or chicken (stick with grilled, pan-seared, or roasted). Ask for ¼ to ⅓ pound (4–6 ounces)—they will weigh it for you. Walk it home. Open it. Heat it. Eat it. Voilà! You've just cooked, my friend.*

Urban Recap

Be prepared at home with healthy snacks; avoid loading your kitchen up with foods you can't just eat one of; and learn some quick ways to prepare really yummy quick dinners so you can "cook" even when you're exhausted.

Up Next

Just like being prepared with food at home, you want your body to be prepared to get you through each day. Most people think they mess up at night, but they really mess up throughout the day by not eating enough of their calories. You don't want to leave yourself starving at night, because you make poor choices when you're starving. Avoiding this means laying the groundwork. Breakfast truly is the most important meal of the day, which makes the next chapter one of the most important of the book.

CHAPTER 7

It All Falls Apart at 4:00 p.m.—
So Build a Good Foundation
with Breakfast and Lunch

Laura, 5'6", generally healthy eater and exercise enthusiast

Urban Challenge
Laura ate well and hit the gym at least five times every week, so she was confused when she gained 10 pounds in just six months. Laura wouldn't eat much during the day, maybe 600 calories. She usually had just veggies and a small amount of protein, and she intentionally restricted her starch intake, avoiding breads and cereals. When she got home she would eat a small dinner. But around 8:00 p.m. she'd be sitting in front of the television and end up eating about 1000 calories, usually carbohydrates and sweets. Popcorn and Tootsie Rolls were always on hand. She was convinced she had no willpower and thought she was addicted to sugar.

Urban Surprise
Laura didn't have any kind of addiction at all. She was depriving her-self all day of anything satisfying in her effort to "eat well." She was essentially starving herself, but thinking she was doing the right thing. She wasn't overeating so much as she wasn't pacing herself. She was

using the cash-and-spend mentality—hoarding her food till the end of the day and mindlessly blowing it all on large amounts.

Urban Insight

Laura was simply too good during the day. She was so obsessed with what went in her mouth before 4:00 p.m. that her evenings crumbled. Laura's first step was to make sure she ate two solid square meals a day and a snack before 4:00 p.m. She always included protein, fat, and carbs in every meal and consumed 1000 calories before her evening even began. She was no longer ravenous by the time she got home and so she ate a nice even 500–600 calorie meal. She realized she wasn't really addicted to sugar and was able to shed the weight she'd gained and keep it off.

Spread Out Your Calories

Did your mother ever tell you that nothing really good happens after midnight? Well, a similar principle applies to weight loss, but the witching hour for dieting is more like 4:00 p.m. And do you know why? Because most people shoot themselves in the foot long before the clock strikes 4:00 p.m. What you eat early in the day is critical to losing weight because you need to eat enough. Willpower during the day isn't the problem; it's the fact that you're setting yourself up for failure at night.

In their attempts to lose weight, many people under-eat during the day to save calories. They may also think they do well with their breakfast and lunch, are fine with not eating much during the day, and struggle at night. Guess what? They're wrong. We call those "famous last words." You screw up at night precisely because your breakfasts and lunches weren't fine—they were too small and not satisfying. Who can resist eating anything in sight or gorging on a huge dinner after not eating all day? The better—and only effective—option is to eat properly during the day (watching portions, not starving, and including protein, fat, and color in each meal) and cut back at dinner so you don't set yourself up for hunger.

URBAN INSIGHT: A busy work day and stress can sometimes distract you during the day and make you forget to, or choose not to, eat. Once you wind down, you'll blow the diet because hunger will take control of your willpower. If it doesn't get you that night, you'll chow big time the following morning.

If you're hungry, you feel deprived, and you most likely didn't have the right lunch, the right snacks, and most important, the right breakfast, you're going to destroy your calorie budget. Breakfast can't be yogurt, fruit, or egg whites alone. It needs to be breakfast. Check again and commit to memory how many calories you should be eating at breakfast. They should equal roughly 25 percent of your daily intake.

Your mother was right about a bunch of other things as well: You should wear clean underwear in case a bus hits you, you are the company you keep, and in fact breakfast is the most important meal of the day. Spending your calories while you're in control is important, since sanity goes out the window when you are super hungry. Make sure your breakfast is a nice foundation for the day.

Why You Need to Lay the Right Foundation

When you starve yourself, your metabolism slows down. If you don't eat enough food to get your system moving, your body learns to adjust and make do with what you give it. If you lose your job and less income is coming into the house, you (hopefully) spend less. You'll cut down on shoes, a personal trainer, or going out to dinner. If you make less, you spend less. Similarly, if you take in fewer calories, your body will learn to expend fewer calories. That's great if you're on a desert island with no food, but not so good if you're in the city, working and being social. In fact, it's the exact opposite of what you want it to do when you're trying to lose weight. If you chronically under-eat, you'll slow your metabolism down, making it more difficult to lose weight.

You've probably heard the term "resting metabolic rate." It's the amount of calories your body needs to function at rest. If you starve yourself, your body knows what you're doing; it'll figure it out and make adjustments to make do with less. It will learn to conserve the food you do give it and become more efficient, which is the very opposite of what you want to happen when you are trying to shed some weight. The damage you do daily will become long-term damage and will make your weight loss a near impossibility. You're built to survive.

Don't cheat the system—because the system is you. You may think eating a smaller breakfast will save you calories, but in fact it will cost you calories. You'll slow your metabolism down and set yourself up to overeat later in the day.

Breakfast of Champions

A proper breakfast is key to losing weight. Skipping or skimping is not good, it's bad. Even though you're rushed, stressed, or whatever, eat—and eat the right amount. Research shows over and over again that breakfast eaters are thinner people. And never mind losing the weight, breakfast is critical for maintenance, too. You won't keep off what you've lost if you skip breakfast.

Unfortunately, you can't say you don't know what to have for breakfast, because we're giving you enough Urban Skinny options to have something different every day of the week. Don't use time as an excuse. Nobody's asking you to whip up eggs Benedict; some of these options can be grabbed and eaten in minutes.

Note: None of these breakfast options include buttered toast, but if you want it—have it. Just make sure you account for it. One tablespoon of butter is 100 calories. Even better, one tablespoon of whipped butter is 60 calories.

300-calorie breakfasts:

- ☐ 1 slice whole-wheat toast and 1 tablespoon peanut butter, with either a small banana or a small skim cappuccino
- ☐ homemade egg sandwich made with a whole-wheat English muffin and 1 egg, plus 1 cup of berries

- ☐ deli option: English muffin, one egg, half a cup of berries
- ☐ whole-grain cereal (100 calories worth), ½ cup skim milk, ½ cup berries, 2 tablespoons chopped almonds
- ☐ Starbucks yogurt parfait
- ☐ small shake from the gym—with 1 scoop protein powder, skim milk, and 1 scoop berries or ½ banana
- ☐ Quaker Weight Control oatmeal packet made with skim milk, 2 tablespoons sliced almonds
- ☐ homemade egg-white omelet—4 egg whites, 1 ounce cheese, veggies, whole-wheat English muffin
- ☐ deli/restaurant choice—egg whites with veggies and cheese (ask them to cook with spray, not oil), 1 slice whole-wheat toast
- ☐ 2 poached or hard-boiled eggs, 1 slice whole-wheat toast, ½ cup berries
- ☐ ½ bagel topped with 1 tablespoon cream cheese, small OJ (4 ounces)
- ☐ 1 glazed donut, small skim cappuccino
- ☐ 1 cup nonfat cottage cheese, 2 tablespoons nuts, ½ cup fruit
- ☐ Balance bar and 1 piece of fruit

350-calorie breakfasts:

- ☐ 1 slice whole-grain or cinnamon-raisin toast, 1½ tablespoons peanut butter, and a small banana
- ☐ Quaker Weight Control oatmeal packet made with skim milk, 2 tablespoons sliced almonds, and 2 tablespoons raisins or ½ banana
- ☐ egg sandwich made with a whole-wheat English muffin, 1 egg, and ½ ounce cheese, plus 1 cup berries
- ☐ deli option—English muffin, 1 egg, 1 cup berries

- whole-grain cereal (150 calories worth), ½ cup skim milk, ½ cup berries, 2 tablespoons chopped almonds
- Starbucks reduced-fat coffee cake and cup of coffee
- small shake from the gym—with 1 scoop protein powder, skim milk, ½ cup yogurt, and 1 fruit
- homemade egg-white omelet—4 egg whites, 1 ounce cheese, veggies, whole-wheat English muffin, ½ cup fruit
- deli omelet—egg whites with veggies, English muffin
- 2 poached or hard-boiled eggs, whole-wheat English muffin, 1 cup berries
- 1 cake donut, small skim cappuccino
- 1 cup nonfat cottage cheese, 2 tablespoons nuts, 1 cup fruit
- Balance bar and 6 ounces low-fat yogurt

> **Yogurt added to shakes should be yogurt, not frozen yogurt, and "bagels scooped" means dig out the insides of the bagel and only eat the outer part!**

400-calorie breakfasts:

- whole-wheat English muffin, 1½ tablespoons peanut butter, and a small banana
- homemade egg sandwich made with whole-wheat English muffin, 1 egg, and 1 ounce cheese, plus 1 cup of berries
- Quaker Weight Control oatmeal packet made with skim milk, 2 tablespoons sliced almonds, 2 tablespoons raisins
- deli option—English muffin, 1 egg, 1 slice cheese, 1 cup of berries
- whole-grain cereal (200 calories worth), ½ cup skim milk, ½ cup berries, 2 tablespoons chopped almonds
- Starbucks yogurt parfait and tall skim cappuccino
- small shake from the gym—with 1 scoop protein powder, skim milk, ½ cup yogurt, and 2 fruits

- ☐ homemade egg-white omelet—4 egg whites, 1 ounce cheese, veggies, whole-wheat English muffin, 1 cup fruit
- ☐ deli omelet—egg whites with veggies, 2 thin slices cheese, English muffin
- ☐ 2 poached or hard-boiled eggs, 2 slices whole-wheat toast, ½ cup berries
- ☐ 1 bagel with the inside scooped out, topped with 2 table-spoons cream cheese
- ☐ jelly or Boston cream donut, small skim cappuccino
- ☐ 1 cup nonfat cottage cheese, 3 tablespoons nuts, 1 cup fruit

450-calorie breakfasts:

- ☐ whole-wheat English muffin, 2 tablespoons peanut butter, and a small banana
- ☐ homemade egg sandwich—2 slices whole-wheat bread, 1 egg, 1 ounce cheese, plus 1 cup of berries
- ☐ 2 Quaker Weight Control oatmeal packets made with water, 2 tablespoons sliced almonds, 2 tablespoons raisins
- ☐ deli option—2 slices whole-wheat toast, 1 egg, 1 slice cheese, 1 cup of berries
- ☐ whole-grain cereal (200 calories worth), 1 cup skim milk, ½ cup berries, 2 tablespoons chopped almonds
- ☐ Starbucks reduced-fat coffee cake and tall skim cappuccino
- ☐ medium shake from the gym—with 2 scoops protein powder, skim milk, ½ cup yogurt, and 2 fruits
- ☐ homemade egg-white omelet—6 egg whites, 1 ounce cheese, veggies, whole-wheat English muffin, 1 cup fruit
- ☐ deli omelet—egg whites with veggies and 2 thin slices cheese, English muffin, ½ cup fruit

- ☐ 1 bagel scooped, topped with 2 tablespoons cream cheese, small OJ (4–6 ounces)
- ☐ 2 poached or hard-boiled eggs, 2 slices whole-wheat toast, 1 cup berries
- ☐ jelly or Boston cream donut, medium skim cappuccino
- ☐ 1 cup nonfat cottage cheese, 2 tablespoons nuts, 1 cup fruit, 1 slice whole-wheat toast

500-calorie breakfasts:

- ☐ 2 slices whole-wheat toast, 2 tablespoons peanut butter, small banana
- ☐ homemade egg sandwich—2 slices whole-wheat bread, 2 eggs, 1 ounce cheese, ½ cup berries
- ☐ 2 Quaker Weight Control oatmeal packets made with hot water, 2 tablespoons sliced almonds, 3 tablespoons raisins
- ☐ deli option—2 slices whole-wheat toast, 2 eggs, 1 cup berries
- ☐ whole-grain cereal (250 calories worth), 1 cup skim milk, ½ cup berries, 2 tablespoons chopped almonds
- ☐ Starbucks reduced-fat coffee cake and grande skim latte
- ☐ large shake from the gym—with 2 scoops protein powder, skim milk, ½ cup yogurt, and 2 fruits
- ☐ homemade egg-white omelet—6 egg whites, 1 ounce cheese, veggies, 2 slices whole-wheat toast, 1 cup fruit
- ☐ deli omelet—egg whites with veggies, 2 thin slices cheese, English muffin, 1 cup fruit
- ☐ 2 poached or hard-boiled eggs, 2 slices whole-wheat toast, 6 ounces nonfat yogurt
- ☐ 1 bagel topped with 2 tablespoons cream cheese
- ☐ 2 glazed donuts or 1 reduced-fat muffin, small skim cappuccino

□ 1 cup nonfat cottage cheese, 2 tablespoons nuts, 1 cup fruit, whole-wheat English muffin

550-calorie breakfasts:

□ 2 slices whole-wheat toast, 2 tablespoons peanut butter, large banana

□ homemade egg sandwich—2 slices whole-wheat bread, 2 eggs, 1 ounce cheese, 1 cup berries

□ 2 Quaker Weight Control oatmeal packets made with skim milk, 2 tablespoons sliced almonds, 2 tablespoons raisins

> **When you're ordering takeout or a deli breakfast, nobody will likely measure your food—so approximate. For example, two thin slices of cheese is the same as one ounce of cheese, which is 100 calories.**

□ deli option—2 slices whole-wheat toast, 2 eggs, 1 slice cheese, 1 cup berries

□ whole-grain cereal (250 calories worth), 1 cup skim milk, 1 cup berries, 2 tablespoons chopped almonds

□ Starbucks reduced-fat coffee cake and venti skim latte

□ large shake from the gym—2 scoops protein powder, skim milk, 1 cup yogurt, and 2 fruits

□ homemade egg-white omelet—6 egg whites, 1½ ounces cheese, veggies, 2 slices whole-wheat toast, 1 cup fruit

□ deli omelet—egg whites with veggies, 2 thin slices cheese, 2 slices whole-wheat toast, 1 cup fruit

□ 2 poached or hard-boiled eggs, 2 slices whole-wheat toast, 1 cup berries, 6 ounces nonfat yogurt

□ 1 bagel topped with 2 tablespoons cream cheese

□ 2 glazed donuts or 1 reduced-fat muffin, medium skim cappuccino

☐ 1 cup nonfat cottage cheese, 2 tablespoons nuts, 1 cup
   fruit, 2 slices whole-wheat toast

Power Snacks

Snacking is a good thing, not a bad thing. Remember that eating every
three to four hours is critical, which is where snacks come in—you don't
want to get too hungry and then "fall off" your plan by gorging out of
starvation. Check the clock, check your eating schedule, and work your
snacks in accordingly. If you get up at 5:00 a.m. and eat before 7:00
a.m., but don't eat lunch until 1:00 p.m., then a morning snack is war-
ranted. If you eat breakfast at 8:30 a.m. at your desk and lunch at noon,
then you don't need a mid-morning snack.

Dinner can get late, so time your mid-afternoon snack as well. A
snack can be dinner's appetite suppressant and prevent overeating.
Avoid saving up all of your calories for one meal at the end of the day.
Don't count on caffeine for the afternoon boost either—energy comes
from food, not coffee. A coffee boost will cause a quick crash later.

100-calorie snacks: mid-a.m. or afternoon

Snacks that include a little protein and fat will keep you satisfied longer.

☐ 1 tablespoon peanut butter (right off the spoon)

☐ 1 tablespoon peanut butter on celery sticks

☐ ½ tablespoon peanut butter on 1 caramel-flavored rice
   cake

☐ ½ tablespoon peanut butter on ½ banana or apple

☐ 20 peanuts or pistachios

☐ 10 peanuts or pistachios and 1 small piece of fruit

☐ 10 walnuts, cashews, or pecan halves

☐ 5 walnuts, cashews, or pecan halves and 1 small piece of
   fruit

☐ 1 ounce of cheese and 1 cup chopped veggies

- ☐ 6 ounces Fage Total 0% yogurt topped with either one tablespoon low-sugar jam or ½ tablespoon honey
- ☐ 1-ounce individual packaged cheese (Cabot, Cracker Barrel, Polly-O, and Horizon brands all have them)
- ☐ Your favorite 100-calorie snack pack (e.g., Nabisco brand)
- ☐ 4-ounce individual pack of cottage cheese (0 or 1% milk fat)
- ☐ 8–10 ounces skim milk
- ☐ 1 small skim latte
- ☐ 1 medium skim cappuccino
- ☐ 1 tall Caffé Vanilla Frappuccino Light Blended Coffee
- ☐ 1 ounce pretzels or baked chips
- ☐ ¼ cup hummus and your favorite veggies
- ☐ 100-calorie snack bag of microwave popcorn
- ☐ 1 packet Quaker Lower Sugar oatmeal

200-calorie snacks: mid-a.m. or afternoon

- ☐ 1 tablespoon peanut butter on 1 slice whole-wheat bread
- ☐ 1 tablespoon peanut butter on 1 graham cracker sheet
- ☐ 2 tablespoons peanut butter on celery sticks
- ☐ 1 tablespoon peanut butter on 1 caramel rice cake topped with ½ sliced banana
- ☐ 1 tablespoon peanut butter on 1 banana or apple
- ☐ 35 peanuts
- ☐ 50 pistachios
- ☐ 1 ounce any type of nuts
- ☐ 20 peanuts or pistachios and 1 piece fruit
- ☐ 20 walnuts, cashews, or pecan halves
- ☐ 10 walnuts, cashews, or pecan halves and 1 small piece of fruit

- ☐ ⅓ cup trail mix
- ☐ 1-ounce box raisins and 10 almonds
- ☐ 6 ounces Fage Total 0% yogurt topped with ¼ cup granola
- ☐ 8 ounces 0 or 1% cottage cheese sprinkled with cinnamon
- ☐ 4-ounce individual pack of cottage cheese (0 or 1% milk fat) and 1 cup fresh fruit
- ☐ 1-ounce individual packaged cheese (Cabot, Cracker Barrel, Polly-O, and Horizon brands all have them) and 1 100-calorie snack pack of crackers
- ☐ 1 100-calorie snack pack of cookies and 8 ounces skim milk
- ☐ 1 medium skim latte and 1 madeleine cookie
- ☐ 2 Oreos and 8 ounces skim milk
- ☐ 1 grande Caffé Vanilla Frappuccino Light Blended Coffee
- ☐ ½ cup hummus and your favorite veggies
- ☐ 200-calorie bag of 94% fat-free microwave popcorn
- ☐ 1 Balance bar
- ☐ 1 ZonePerfect bar
- ☐ 1 Luna bar
- ☐ 1 whole-grain Pop-Tart
- ☐ 200-calorie Quaker Oatmeal Express cup
- ☐ 1 package peanut-butter-and-cheddar-cheese crackers

300-calorie snacks: mid-a.m. or afternoon

- ☐ 1 tablespoon peanut butter on 1 slice whole-wheat bread and 8 ounces skim milk
- ☐ 2 tablespoons peanut butter and 1 tablespoon honey on 1 graham cracker sheet
- ☐ 2 tablespoons peanut butter on 2 caramel rice cakes

☐ 2 tablespoons peanut butter on 1 banana or apple

☐ ⅓ cup (50ish) peanuts

☐ 1 cup in the shell pistachios

☐ 35 peanuts and 1 piece fruit

☐ 30 walnuts, cashews, or pecan halves

☐ 20 walnuts, cashews, or pecan halves and 1 small piece of fruit

☐ ½ cup trail mix

☐ 1-ounce box raisins and 25 almonds

☐ 6 ounces Fage Total 0% yogurt topped with ½ cup granola and 2 tablespoons slivered almonds

☐ 8 ounces 0 or 1% cottage cheese with 1 cup fresh fruit, 1 tablespoon almonds

☐ 1-ounce individual packaged cheese (Cabot, Cracker Barrel, Polly-O, and Horizon brands all have them) and 1 100-calorie snack pack of crackers and 1 piece of fruit

☐ 1 medium skim latte and 1 almond biscotti (Starbucks)

☐ 3 Oreos and 12 ounces skim milk

☐ 1 grande Caffé Vanilla Frappuccino Light Blended Coffee and 1 madeleine cookie

☐ ¼ cup hummus and 1-ounce bag Stacy's pita chips

☐ 1 Balance bar and 1 piece of fruit

☐ 1 ZonePerfect bar and 1 piece of fruit

☐ 1 Luna bar and 1 piece of fruit

☐ 1 Snickers or Twix bar

URBAN INSIGHT: If you want nuts for your snack, stick to the ones in the shell. You have to work to eat them, which stretches out your snack. It takes you longer to eat them that way.

Staying Fueled for Fitness

Snacking is important for keeping fueled and energized throughout the day, but it can also be used strategically when you're working out. The right snack will help you not only "get through" your workout, but actually kick some butt and get to another level. Even if you're not training for the Olympics, you'll want to maximize fuel to boost performance.

Morning Workouts

The food has to not only be digested but absorbed and metabolized into a usable form before your body can convert it to energy. So that high-protein bar you choked down on the way over to the gym—15–20 minutes before you got on the treadmill—will just be burped up during your run. Keep it small. All you need is a quick 50–100 calories before you start to sweat (unless you're doing more than 90 minutes, in which case you will need 200 calories).

Fruit is a great pre-workout snack: It's portable and it helps you reach your fruit and veggie intake! Grab a piece of fruit or a handful of grapes 15 minutes before you hit the gym. You can also try one handful of a cereal such as Cheerios, Kashi Heart to Heart, or Raisin Bran, one sheet of low-fat graham cracker, or a 100-calorie granola bar.

Evening Workouts

Your afternoon snack is ultra-important for energy, and also strategic because you won't finish the workout starving, which as we all know results in a major dinner pig-out. So you'll get a great boost to plow through your workout, but you'll also save yourself from overeating later.

Urban Recap

Stay fueled, keep your energy up, eat every three to four hours, never ever skip breakfast, use snacks strategically for energy, and don't let yourself get hungry.

Up Next

Now that you've got the basics down, you can take care of yourself and manage your weight if all goes as planned. But c'mon, what ever goes as planned? Vacations and all kinds of crazy situations will arise, so you're going to have to know how to wing it in the air and just plain wing it on the ground when life gets in the way.

CHAPTER 8

Taking Flight—
You've Got a Ticket to Fly,
Not Eat

Mala, successful real estate developer, travels often

Urban Challenge

Mala's trips out of the country were every other week and usually lasted four days at a time. She'd always catch the 4:00 p.m. flight on Monday and grab a morning flight home on Friday. The flight times were also meal times, which messed up Mala's eating. In addition, Mala missed her family, which led her to consume more than she would at home. Like many people's, Mala's eating issues were the result of a couple of problems—for her, it was both the inconvenience of travel and its emotional challenges.

Urban Surprise

Mala was always sent to the same places—Costa Rica and Puerto Rico—so she was very familiar with the areas. She knew which restaurants were convenient and she was a regular at certain hotels. The airplanes and the airports, while also familiar, threw her for a loop because she felt since she was on the move she could eat more mindlessly and not blame herself for it.

Urban Insight

Mala started calling the hotel ahead of time and asking that the minibar in her room be cleared out before she arrived so she wasn't tempted by chips and chocolate late at night. On her way to the airport in the afternoon, she snacked on a bag of nuts to cut the hunger. She ate an actual meal on the plane; since she flew first class she always ordered the chicken or shrimp and turned down the cookies and ice cream. Once she arrived, she made a point to phone, text, or e-mail home when she felt lonely, instead of turning to food as a distraction. She also created some consistency by making sure she stayed at the same place in each country. It eased the tension of her crazy schedule and gave her a pattern to follow when ordering at the hotel. Breakfast was always poached eggs, toast, and fresh fruit from room service. On the trip home, she made certain to eat—either before she got on the plane or on the plane—and just to have a light snack at home once she got in. This helped her avoid eating two dinners or gorging once she was in her own kitchen.

Calories Always Count, No Matter Where You Are

You can be a jet-setter and still lose weight. Just remember—you've got a ticket to fly, not to eat. Travel does not have to harpoon your dieting efforts.

If you are a true jet-setter, you likely travel all the time, whether for business or to some steamy destination with your latest beau. Even so, Urban Skinny rules always apply, even on the road. Don't get a "road-trip" mentality when you fly. College road trips were for binge eating and drinking; civilized grown-up ones in the sky are not. Just because you eat the calories at 30,000 feet doesn't mean they don't count. Rack up frequent flier miles, not calories.

Have a Flight Plan

Business trips and fun trips can be treated somewhat differently when it comes to eating, but no matter where you're flying, don't waste a ton of your calories on airplane food—save them for something yummier. It's not a newsflash; airplane food can be lousy. Even if Charlie Trotter himself is cooking those beef tips with noodles, they're not going to taste as good reheated and served in a foil tray. Eat on a plane, but don't overeat just because it's sitting in front of you. Save any indulgence for the destination.

> **URBAN INSIGHT:** Eat salad first, if you're on an airline that offers a meal. Pre-order a special meal—low calorie or heart healthy. Vegan might not always be low calorie. Skip the dessert; it's probably not worth the calories. Get rid of your tray as soon as possible so you don't pick at what you originally passed on.

Your flight plan for eating varies according to your actual flight plan. Pick a scenario and let's work through your trip.

Stick to Your Meal Pattern

If you're flying during mealtime, you can work your meal in. If you're flying in the middle of the afternoon, don't eat a second lunch. Lunchtime is lunchtime whether you're at your desk, on a layover in the lounge, on the plane, or at the gate. So schedule your food accordingly, and keep your afternoon snack handy. When people get out of their normal routine they panic. Don't panic. Grab a small sandwich, get a salad, eat at the gate or on the plane—but keep to your schedule. A flight to LA or Cabo can still be a weight-loss day.

Keep Things Simple

If you have a 1:30 p.m. flight, but you usually eat at noon, eat at noon. Use the time you're waiting for your flight and make your meal a proper Urban Skinny one. Unless you're flying out of some remote airport like Patriot Hills Antarctica (which is just a slab of ice), you'll be surprised by the food now available at airports. JetBlue's T5 terminal at JFK has a sushi restaurant and a little general store that sells fresh fruit, yogurt, bars, and turkey sandwiches on whole grain, leaving no room for the excuse "I was in an airport." And you can buy something for your flight if you want to skip the airplane food.

URBAN INSIGHT: When in doubt, grab a basic slice of pizza with cheese and veggies and as thin a crust as is available. It's generally a solid 500 calories and it will fill you up.

Overnight Travel

You don't normally eat when you sleep, do you? Just in case you haven't learned yet, if you follow Urban Skinny, you're likely eating every three to four hours. But if you're on an overnight flight to Europe, you're supposed to be sleeping, not eating. Don't laugh—many people think they should eat every three to four hours even on an overnight flight (yes, clients have actually asked if they should). Obviously, if you were home, you'd be sleeping, not eating. Don't fall out of your Urban Skinny food routine. In fact, on overnight flights, eat dinner before you fly, and tell the flight attendant not to serve you until he or she wakes you up for breakfast. You avoid a sleep interruption and calorie-wasting temptation. If you already ate dinner and they try to serve you dinner, remember this: It's a free world, you can say no. You wouldn't eat two dinners at home, would you? Why would you eat twice just because you are flying to Rome?

Jet Lag and Eating

Jet lag makes people feel very tired and out of sorts, which often leads to overeating. Employ whatever tricks you can to get on the local schedule as quickly as possible so you can get your eating schedule on track, too. Drink lots of water, sleep at night (not during the day), and don't eat extra meals. Eat breakfast, lunch, snack, and dinner at the local times, no matter where you are.

URBAN INSIGHT: If the airport offers you nothing but fast food, be a kid again and order the kid-size food. McDonald's, for example, offers a four-pack chicken nugget Happy Meal that's less than 450 calories, including the fries. Choose the diet soda. If you get barbecue or honey mustard sauce remember to dip, not dunk. If you're craving the burger, the cheeseburger-and-fries option is just over 500 calories. McDonald's offers salads, too, with dressing on the side. Think small—no big-size anything or your butt will reflect your order.

The Layover or Delay

There's more to life than the airport lounge. Most of us find ourselves at the bar drinking d-list wine, eating a giant plate of waffle fries or some over-touched bowl of bar mix. You can have your cocktail if you work it into your plan, but don't think the only way to pass time is to drink or eat. These days many airport terminals have spas—you can get a manicure, pedicure, or massage. Bookstores are great to kill some time, or leave your bag in the lounge locker and power walk the terminal. Or do some shopping (or just window-shopping if you're not flush with cash). Have you ever been to Heathrow? It's a shopper's paradise—and it's duty free *and* calorie free!

Stick to the Rules

"Bring your own" used to be the best option when flying, but gourmet is making its way both on the plane and at the gate. Now, if you like to pack your own food and it helps you stay on track, fine—go for it. But you can wing the airport eating, just like you do at any restaurant, by sticking to what you've learned about ordering—sauces and dressings on the side, small portions, and do your best to measure. Just because you're in a rush doesn't mean you get fried crap. It takes just as long to order high-calorie fried as it does a turkey sandwich on whole wheat. You get frustrated paying for extra baggage; how irritating will it be when the extra baggage is on your thighs?

> URBAN INSIGHT: Hydrate—it helps with jet lag and cuts the bloat. Airline food is salty and generally low in nutritional value. Flying makes you feel puffy. Don't step on the scale the day you get home from a trip; you'll be discouraged.

Have a Food Itinerary

Even with all your good intentions, travel these days is unpredictable and can throw off the best of schedules. Keep a small bag of nuts or dried fruit or a nutrition or health bar on hand just in case you get stuck. Pack a snack just like you pack your passport. By snack, we mean a couple hundred calories, not enough to feed the entire row. Airport boredom shouldn't become airport binging. Bring a book or your knitting to keep your hands busy, because after six hours on the runway you'll want to hit your entire bag of food tricks.

> URBAN INSIGHT: In coach you may have less legroom, but you may also have less calories. Here's why: no warm nuts, no unlimited booze, and you don't spend any calories just smelling those freshly baked cookies they're having at the front of the plane. But, be mindful—that big, thick slab of pizza-like food or the fake-meat sandwich, the mini chocolate bar, the chips, and the carrots with dip can add up, so pick and choose.

The bottom line in the air, like anywhere, is to follow the Urban Skinny rules. Count your calories, keep your log, don't waste your calories on bad choices, and remember every calorie counts—even on a plane!

Business Trips

Whether you're taking your annual trip to Asia or a last-minute trip to deal with a client crisis in Kansas, a business trip is your job, not a vacation. It's just another Wednesday, not a celebration or a special occasion. So eat like it's just another Wednesday. Order food like you—not the company expense account—are paying for it, and avoid the free-food mentality that suggests more is better. Only the check is taken care of. The calorie surplus is still your problem, not the company's.

Know Your Food Territory

If you're going somewhere you've been before, it's usually easier to plan your food strategy. You know the restaurants, you know the safe orders, and you know the portion sizes. If you're going somewhere unfamiliar, follow the rules in the restaurant chapter; do your homework like usual and know in advance what you're ordering by checking the menu online if you can. If you have no control and a local is taking you out, watch your portions. If your local client asks where you want to eat, follow our advice: Take control. Tell them you'd prefer sushi or fish, safe options for Urban Skinny.

Room Service

There are a few tricks for room service at hotels, whether you're on a business or pleasure trip.

First of all, don't look at the menu if it's late; you've just traveled for eight hours and you're cranky. Just dial room service and ask for a simple salad with chicken, a piece of grilled fish and a salad, or a basic grilled chicken sandwich. Don't tempt yourself and end up eating a three-course meal at midnight. Here are a few more tips to help keep you on track:

- Spa cuisine is offered at a lot of upscale hotels, so when you're awake and fresh, check for heart-healthy options for the following nights.

- Just because you're eating in your room doesn't mean your restaurant rules don't apply. Order mindfully.

- When it comes to breakfast, stick with a bowl of oatmeal, a poached egg or an egg-white omelet, whole-wheat toast and peanut butter, or whole-grain cold cereal and fruit with skim milk. Almost any breakfast option you would make at home you can have at a hotel, and room service will almost always accommodate a special order, so ask for it. Choose from your list of calorie-portioned breakfast picks and stay on track. Again, it's just another day, so just another breakfast—no need to celebrate over Belgian waffles with sausage on the side just because you're making a sales call in Ohio.

Vacation Planning

If it's a once-in-a-lifetime trip, your honeymoon, or some other monumental event (meaning not your annual trip to South Beach), you may want to consider shooting for maintenance—holding on to your weight loss so far, rather than trying to lose more—while you're away. If you gain two pounds while you're gone, don't totally freak out—when you're back you can pick up where you left off and lose it again.

Even on a maintenance plan you'll face some challenges. You might have that extra cocktail or two, or half a dessert. You might have both your starch and your wine at one sitting. Those little shifts in your behavior are fine; they are maintenance-type moves. But that doesn't mean that pigging out while you're away is okay. Maintenance means following the rules, but a little less rigidly. You're only away for a week or two—eating to maintain means adding 200–300 calories to your diet each day. Don't eat to gain. Don't throw all the hard work out the window, but enjoy your trip. Sample the local fare and absorb the culture.

If your goal is to bring home a snow-globe souvenir but a few less pounds, try to stay in calorie-check. While you're away, you're going to have to stick to your calorie count; follow your Urban Skinny plan and that may be easy enough. You might find it's not as much about good nutrition on the trip, but it has to be about calories. Don't beat yourself up if you

> You'd have to eat an extra 3500 calories in order to gain one pound, so even if you eat an extra 200 a day while you're away, you won't move the scale.

have too many fatty foods, but keep it within your calorie count and you won't gain. If sticking to 1500 calories a day helped you lose pounds at home, 1500 calories a day will cause weight loss while in Buenos Aires, too. The calorie formula doesn't change with the time zone. It's only seven days—you can temporarily eat some junk . . . just don't overeat. Get through the vacation with not-so-hot food picks, but that's not a forever way to eat.

Now, on vacation your schedule may shift along with your attitude. You might sleep a little later or linger out a little longer at night, so your breakfast-lunch-dinner schedule might get a little warped. Your Urban Skinny routine might shift. That's okay. If you have brunch at 11:00 a.m. and a snack in the afternoon, followed by a late dinner, that's okay.

Just be strategic about it. If one day you treat yourself at breakfast to a famous French pastry, don't later have cheese and an aperitif as your snack. If you're in Paris for six days, you have time to spread out the indulgence; you don't have to cram it all into one day. The same rule applies to a resort or cruise with a buffet—you've got a week in the sand and sun, so try one thing each day, not all things in one day. And on those all-inclusives, don't work to get your money's worth. The price you pay when you get home will be in weight gain.

Urban Myth: *If you're on a tropical beach vacation, you should indulge in all the drinks and food offered.*

Urban Skinny: *You need to earn the right to sit in a lounge chair all day in your new bikini; earn it by going to the gym. Remember when you're working sixty hours a week and you don't have time for the gym? Well, you've got nothing but time in the Caymans. And since you spend your city days on the treadmill, try something new—investigate beach walks or trails around your hotel; most nice hotels have jogging maps. Or try a sunrise yoga or post-beach vinyasa.*

URBAN INSIGHT: By the pool, order a non-frozen rum drink with fruit juices instead of the piña coladas. You'll only consume 250 calories versus an artery-clogging cocktail made with cream!

Urban Skinny Trips

Avoid fat-farm starvation vacations—you can't accomplish a lifelong goal in just a week or two. Remember those trips are designed for quick results, not necessarily permanent ones. When you get back, you're starting in a hole. The 500 calories a day you were placed on at the "spa" will arguably just ensure that your metabolism will be out of whack. You'll gain the weight back. Detox diets create unrealistic goals and are nothing but starvation.

The only detox you should be doing is a purge from fad diets. Instead, take an active trip. They're great for everyone, but especially good if you're single because your travel companions come with the trip. If you want to go to Italy, don't eat your way through the country, climb through it: Plan a trek in the Dolomites with an organized group. Ski the Alps, do an adventure trip in New Zealand, or sign up for a yoga retreat. At least you're working for your dinner when you're active all day. If you look "vacation" up in the dictionary, the definition isn't "piña coladas poolside."

Urban Myth: *You'll gain weight on a European vacation.*

Urban Skinny: *You're walking for hours every day sightseeing, which helps balance out your calorie intake. If you're in Italy, the gelato is a tiny serving, making it a perfect afternoon snack. In France, the portions are smaller than in the States, and in Greece fish is an option everywhere. Stick to your rules and enjoy the culture and you'll be fine.*

Just remember, a holiday is about vacation, chilling, relaxing, and sleeping in. Only certain trips are all about the cuisine. Enjoy a massage, take in a sunset, make a vacation enjoyable in other ways, because if you overeat, the return to reality will be extra miserable.

Urban Myth: *A trip to Aspen is a healthy trip because you're skiing.*

Urban Skinny: *With downhill skiing your movement might be in fifteen-minute increments. You're not "skiing" for eight hours—warm-up, chairlift, lunch, and après-ski take time—so fuel accordingly, not like you're carb-loading for an Olympic slalom race.*

Urban Recap

Eat what you need to eat on a plane if it's mealtime, but don't overeat. Treat a business trip like any other day at work, except you're in a different city. And if you're on vacation, either plan to maintain, not lose, or work out to earn your beach time.

Up Next

Airports and planes aren't the only hurdles you'll face. Sometimes you'll need to wing it at home and work as well. The next chapter will help you do just that and stay on track. All the planning in the world could fall apart when strange situations arise, so have a plan B, or be ready to wing it. Don't cry into your bubbly when your schedule changes. Unexpected meetings, dates, or traffic jams aren't hand-engraved invitations to chow down because you got thrown for a loop. Be prepared to throw your preparation out the window and still lose weight.

CHAPTER 9

Be Street Smart—
Always Have a Plan B

Doreen started Urban Skinny while she was in the middle of a divorce. She had let her weight creep up to 180 pounds, even though she was just 5'4". She wanted to be 140 pounds.

Urban Challenge

Doreen is a single mom and a highly successful corporate lawyer. Some days her son would throw a major temper tantrum, and by the time she got him calmed down and out the door, there was no time for breakfast. Her son developed asthma and frequently had to be rushed to the emergency room. As a result of the divorce, he often had bad dreams at night, and so she was often exhausted. Lunch occasionally got disrupted by emergency overseas conference calls. And as if life hadn't already thrown her enough curve balls, Doreen's newly renovated apartment got visited by bedbugs.

Urban Surprise

Doreen could chart out a plan for weight loss easily enough. She understood the logic, science, and strategy behind the process, and had the drive and motivation to follow a plan to get her weight on track. The problem: Nothing ever went as planned for Doreen.

Urban Insight

Doreen's Urban Skinny planning started not only with having a plan, but with having a plan B. If she missed the healthy pre-planned breakfast, plan B was an on-the-go glazed donut and a banana. The calories were in check and she was able to ensure she ate breakfast. Egg whites and toast from the deli were another breakfast back-up, and there was a place by her son's school that made them quickly, so she didn't lose too much time on the run. Lunch's plan B required recruits. Doreen's assistant was given three safe takeout picks, and she was to make sure one of them was on Doreen's desk at lunchtime even if Doreen was on a call. The food was dropped in front of her so she could eat while she worked.

Plan B for working out was easy: Doreen walked the one and a half miles home from work every day. Plan A was the gym. If she couldn't walk (Plan B), at the very least, she popped an exercise DVD in and did something in the living room. The point: Always have a back-up so there's no excuse. It gave her a 30-minute cardio boost and a chance to decompress so she didn't go home and overeat out of frustration and stress. Low-calorie frozen dinners became Doreen's go-to. She also had her sushi place programmed into her cell phone. She would call before she finished her walk home so her healthy, calories-in-check option arrived home just after she did. There was little room left for error or careless ordering.

Urban Success

Doreen lost 30 pounds. She wasn't skipping meals because she had both a plan and a back-up plan. Doreen learned some tricks and was able to eat on a regular schedule and stick within her calorie recommendation. She still has days that are challenging, but she is on her way to hitting her weight goal.

Expect the Unexpected

Nobody said life was easy—things happen and we all face challenges. Not letting those challenges impair your weight-loss quest is critical.

When well-laid plans don't go our way we often say, "See, I can't lose weight; life's too stressful." But one situation, one meal, one sugary snack does not have to screw up your whole day. That's one of the most valuable lessons you can learn from Urban Skinny.

You're inevitably going to face a few hiccups along the way, but make sure you separate the hiccups from the major roadblocks. If something really bad impacts your life, priorities like diet and exercise often go on the back burner. But this chapter isn't about dealing with those kinds of problems; instead it tackles the little things that don't ruin your life but definitely complicate your day. You have to learn how to distinguish between the two, stay consistent and on track, and not throw in the food towel just because you broke your heel on the way to work.

Part of the Urban Skinny strategy, and your key to success, is having a back-up plan—a plan B for every situation. That's because you can't let a mishap in the middle of the day, or one moment of weakness in your eating, derail a day or a week's worth of hard work. If you eat too much at lunch, tweak your plan and eat less at dinner. Don't say "I'll start again tomorrow" and eat more. If you get stuck in a situation, have a meal plan backup and roll with it. You can't control everything, but by having a plan B, you can avoid getting into a food jam that sets you up to make bad choices.

> **It Can't Be Said Enough**
> - **There are no good or bad foods—rather than skip breakfast because you missed the subway, a 200-calorie donut will do in a pinch so you can stay on track.**
> - **One food cannot blow your healthy eating plan.**
> - **Portion control is always key.**

Urban Skinny Scenarios That Require a Plan B

Never say f@$% it, never panic, and never throw in the towel. There's always a way to get back on track. No day is ever shot over one misstep.

Morning Mix-Ups

You may have the best intentions for a healthy breakfast, and then your day gets off to a bad start. Of course that veggie omelet is not going to happen on these days, but you should never skip breakfast, so kick into plan B:

- ☐ Keep whole-wheat English muffins in the freezer and a jar of peanut butter in case you need an on-the-go, easy-to-make alternative.

- ☐ A very quick pit stop at the coffee cart: A glazed donut is 200 calories and saves you from skipping breakfast, or grab the buttered roll over the bagel and cream cheese— it's half the calories.

- ☐ A nutrition bar and a skim latte are quick.

- ☐ Dunkin' Donuts, Starbucks, and McDonald's have lo-cal options for on-the-go as well.

Meeting Marathon

Meetings are often beyond your control and can really derail your best diet intentions. For starters, if you're in a morning meeting and the muffin tray arrives, don't look at the meeting as an invite to eat an encore breakfast. Instead, grab a coffee and a piece of fruit and step away from the pastries. Or if it's a standing regular meeting, don't eat breakfast at home and have your breakfast during the meeting with everyone else. If you know a meeting is going to last forever, come armed with a snack or maybe suggest ordering lunch in for the group. If you do emerge from a killer long meeting late in the day, foodless and ravenous, head to a safe lunch pick—like your salad bar instead of a den of temptation— or have a bigger lunch than usual and skip the snack. In this situation, chug a big bottle of water to fill the void short-term.

If lunch is provided, choose carefully from the sandwich tray. First pick—turkey; default pick—ham; if-you-must pick—beef. Last-resort sandwich choice is anything mayo-based, like tuna or chicken salad. If mayo-mania is your only pick, grab just half. If you're gravitating toward the cookie tray, one means one (and also means you've had your after-noon snack).

If you have an overseas conference call that just won't end, don't jump overboard. Recruit some help by e-mailing a coworker or your assistant and ask him or her to grab something for you. No skipping meals, no matter what.

Lunch in Limbo

Lunch, like breakfast, is important. If you miss it, and have no plan B, you're going to chow late at night. But don't be rigid. If you truly thought this one time lettuce and tomato wouldn't make your bread soggy, but you made it at home and brought it anyway, switch gears and buy something else. Don't eat something that won't satisfy you. And if you get dragged to a quick off-site sans the brown bag or outside your comfort zone of local lunches, either eat your snack at lunch and eat your lunch at snack time, or buy something before you get back to the office—plan ahead. You will keep yourself fueled and satisfied and not irrationally hungry, grabbing at the closest thing.

Sometimes the trickiest lunch challenges are the ones that hit you afterward—like when you have a lapse in judgment and eat an entire burrito instead of just half. You're going to be full, so skip the afternoon snack and have a lighter dinner. You can still hit your calorie count. Don't assume since you had one moment of weakness you get a special pass to overeat the rest of the day—you don't. Get back on track.

If you squeeze in your workout at lunchtime, just don't let it mess with your eating schedule. Breakfast at 8:00 a.m. and lunch at 2:30 p.m. isn't Urban Skinny–esque. To avoid going too long without eating (and you know by now that's bad), have your afternoon snack at 11:00 a.m. for fuel and to fight hunger, then eat your lunch post-workout.

Afternoon Blunders

If a craving calls, answer the phone. It's better to deal with it in daylight hours while you're mindful than closer to midnight when your judgment is poor. Salt, chocolate, sweet, or crunchy—a craving can be satisfied in two bites. No need for a huge size. Better to grab a small snack-sized bag of chips in the afternoon than eat an entire grocery-sized bag in bed during *Sex and the City* reruns.

Speaking of mid-afternoon snacks, watch out for the office birthday cake. It's always someone's birthday in the office; whether it's yours or someone else's, if you really want the sliver of cake make it your snack. No giant slabs of cake allowed and only indulge on occasion.

If you're having one of those afternoon meetings with a tempting dessert tray, have a plan of attack. One gourmet cookie from the big tray in the conference room with a coffee or tea is allowed as your snack—or take a bar or fruit and nuts in there with you. And if you called the meeting you have the authority to arrange for something healthier, like a veggie or fruit platter.

If you forgot your snack or your desk-drawer snacks are drained by mooching coworkers, run out if you can and refill the bar drawer. If the vending machine is your last-ditch option, grab the nuts, trail mix, or granola bar. Otherwise, pick any snack that fits into your calorie budget. And in warm weather, when snack bars may melt, switch to nuts or non-coated bars.

End-of-Day Fiascos

So, you've managed to stick with your plan all day, and then you're invited to last-minute cocktails with clients, friends, or a hot dude. You don't have to say no and sadly slink home. Have one and run, or just take it slowly so you don't order more, and when you eat dinner, shave a smidge off of your dinner food calories. And remember to order one of your lower-calorie drink options.

URBAN INSIGHT: Eating at night isn't a problem; overeating at night is. Make yourself a simple dinner rather than going to bed hungry. It'll save you a failed start when you wake up starving, causing you to overeat at breakfast. The mindset of "no eating after 8:00 p.m." is wrong. If you get home at 9:00 p.m. and you haven't had dinner, by all means eat your dinner. Boil some water and have a cup of flavored tea or unsweetened soda or iced tea. If that's just not cuttin' it, one small apple or a small container of blueberries. One hundred calories of fruit one night won't derail your entire weight-loss effort.

If you're stuck at the office at dinnertime, give in and order dinner at work. You may try to get your work done and eat at home, but if it really looks like you won't be home until 10:00 p.m., then it's better to concede defeat now and choose from one of your solid takeout go-to's. Chances are that the later you wait, the more likely you are to fall off the Urban Skinny wagon. And fall hard, like ordering a giant burrito for dinner when you get home or a cheeseburger and fries—which you don't want to eat at midnight, if at all. If you simply can't avoid a really late-night meal, social or otherwise, around 5:30 p.m. try to grab a simple veggie salad with a drizzle of dressing to carry you through so you don't pig out when you get seated.

Wacky Weekends

Weekends can easily throw off your normal eating routine—you sleep in late, you hit the gym, you eat brunch. People tend to get a bit lost on the weekend because their schedules change. You can stay on track by still sticking to a schedule; just make a weekend version. Have fruit pre-workout, then combine breakfast and lunch into a brunch. Make sure you have an afternoon snack so you don't eat one big meal early and nothing again until 8:00 p.m. You still want to spread out the fuel throughout the day.

If you decide to go to the movies during your regular mealtime, just bring a snack with you. Even though you used to be mortified when your dad air popped popcorn at home and made you take it with you, the Urban Skinny–ite can happily strut into a theater armed with snacks or food that coordinates with what you'd be eating at that time of day. If buying popcorn is an essential part of your moviegoing experience, a small is about 400 calories, which makes a handy lunch.

If you're invited to a dinner party you're in the hot seat, because you can't pick the menu, nor can you insult the host by being high maintenance. If a plate is being put in front of you, or worse yet, multiple courses are being served, employ your well-tuned portion-control skills—big time. Taste everything, but eat small amounts and leave food on your plate. Don't insult the chef by skipping a course. If you have to say anything, just say each thing is good, but that you're getting full. If you really want to overdo it, lay it on thick and ask for the recipe. If wine is being served, an ounce or two at each course is fine.

Virtual Office

If you're a television field producer, reporter, or pharmaceutical rep, or for some other reason don't spend all day at a desk, your eating plans can be a challenge. If this is your every day, then your plan B is really your plan A. Always have a food stash in your bag or car. Nuts, bars, peanut butter, water, fruit—you have to load up. Your bag is your desk drawer. Also pack a sandwich; it will travel well and ensures you're always prepared. If food is being served on location, again stick to the smart choices and watch the portion control. Be extra versed on what's in your territory; always learn your fast foods and what's available. If you're on the lookout for markets, bring a groovy-looking lunch-sized cooler bag so you can keep some veggies, yogurt, or other fresh items on hand. And your food won't get crushed in your bag.

Under the Weather

It can be tougher to follow your usual meal plan when you're home sick, because you simply don't feel like eating the same things—especially if you have an upset stomach.

If you're home with the sniffles or a touch of the flu (nothing life or death), the last thing you probably want is a giant salad. Soup is a good choice because it makes you feel good, and if it's not cream-based it's usually low in calories. If you really don't feel like eating, don't stress; you can't force food in just because you're trying to stick to a schedule. Try not to chug a gallon of OJ—maybe stick to a glass and a vitamin C tablet. Water, tea, chicken broth, and sugar-free ginger ale are good options when you're trying to load up on fluids. Unless your doctor writes you a scrip for a tub of ice cream, don't use being sick as an excuse to self-soothe and overindulge.

Urban Recap

Be prepared in case you need to wing it, have a plan-B approach to every situation, and don't use a bump in the road as a reason to eat.

Up Next

If something bad happens and you turn to food, guess what—you've created a second problem for yourself. Perhaps you lost your job, but now you're unemployed *and* overweight. There are ways to deal with life's big issues and strategies to avoid using food as the coping mechanism.

CHAPTER 10

Now You Have
Two Problems—
Keeping Emotional Eating at Bay

Suzanne, successful creative type, 38 years old, single, both parents deceased, strained relationship with her brother

Urban Challenge
Suzanne has struggled with her weight since college. She's a binge eater who uses food to cope with daily problems as well as big-picture life issues. She turns to food not only when she's feeling unhappy with her life, but even when her poker game is going poorly.

Urban Surprise
Suzanne has some self-awareness. She's been seeing a therapist for years to help her deal with life, but the two of them never really focused on how her problems relate to food.

Urban Insight
Organizing her eating proved to be extremely helpful for Suzanne's weight-loss efforts. She got on a meal schedule, and she treats it as seriously as she would a job. She sticks to it and never deviates, no matter how she feels. She eats very consciously and is never left hungry or unsatisfied. Suzanne never cooks. She's super social and eats out

with friends four times a week; she's learned how to master the menu. Other nights, she grabs a healthy pre-made pick from the grocery store or sticks to sushi or a salad. She's lost 68 pounds.

One Problem Is Enough

We all face challenges. Nobody's life is perfect (if someone tells you theirs is, they're lying). The same stuff happens to all of us—life's little (and big) upsets are a constant. What sets us apart is how we handle the ups and downs we're dealt. Even if you don't consider yourself an emotional eater, or you don't think it's your biggest weight-loss issue, you'll still likely identify with this chapter if weight is a challenge in your life. In fact, you might even be unaware of the role food plays in your life when you're under stress.

Stressful situations are everywhere: losing a job, getting dumped by a boyfriend, racking up the credit card bills, getting divorced, or dealing with ailing relatives. Even good things like buying a house or starting a great new job can cause major amounts of stress and anxiety. But if you let your stresses take themselves out on your eating habits, then guess what? Now you have two problems: You're overweight and out of a job. Or you're overweight and you've been dumped. Would you rather be just lonely, or lonely and bigger than you used to be?

Coping Mechanisms Should Never Be Edible

People cope in different ways when things get rough. Some people drink, some people smoke or do drugs, and some people exercise more. There are those who meditate, seek out a shrink, or stay inside and become antisocial. An overwhelming number of people, however, console themselves with food. A lot of people turn to food because it's very readily available and obviously eating is socially acceptable. If you're at work and having a bad day, you can't exactly open up your desk drawer and crack a bottle of Scotch, because aside from raising some eyebrows, you'll likely get dragged down to human resources. But on the other hand, if the market tanks and you forgot to switch your position on a stock, walking to the vending machine for some peanut M&M's will go pretty much unnoticed by everyone around you. A massage works great too, but it's unlikely you keep a masseuse in your drawer next to the paper clips.

In times of stress, you're reacting to a situation. You're not in planning mode. You're not processing information. You're simply reacting without thinking. For many people, going into survival mode means turning to old or familiar behaviors, and for many dieters that means eating. It's easy because it's what you know. For people who struggle with their weight, their biggest comfort comes from food. For those who spend their lives dieting, food is often the only answer.

Urban Myth: *Everyone turns to food to deal with stress.*

Urban Skinny: *More often, it's chronic dieters who eat to de-stress, while non-dieters might turn to the gym. Dieters spend a lot of time depriving themselves of their favorite foods, so when they hit a wall they say "screw it" and shove five cookies in with absolutely no thought. When living an Urban Skinny lifestyle you won't be depriving yourself of anything, so you'll be less likely to turn to food for comfort in rough times.*

URBAN INSIGHT: The more desperate you feel to lose weight, the more extreme measures you take, which is what feeds the fad diet market. Fad diets aren't the way to go—in the long term they only cost you pounds.

Avoiding the Real Issue

Nobody likes to feel angry, sad, lonely, bored, or tired, but if you distract yourself from those feelings by eating, you never really figure out why you're feeling any of those crappy things. It's not easy, but you have to make an effort to find a more productive solution or coping mechanism to get through the day; otherwise you'll always use food and you'll always have a weight problem. It's easy to say "don't be sad," but hard to make yourself snap out of it. But if you really want to break a bad habit, you've got to figure out a way to take eating out of the equation. Gaining weight makes your existing problems seem even worse. Extra weight can make you feel hopeless and frustrated, and you'll create more problems for yourself instead of solving the one that made you eat in the first place. Try to stay positive—success stories come from positive thinkers with an ability to envision success.

URBAN INSIGHT: Losing weight makes you feel more confident, but how you look can't be the sole measurement of your worth. Just because you lose weight doesn't mean you'll solve all your other problems. If the underlying problems that caused you to overeat and gain weight still exist, then you could easily gain the weight back.

Get professional help if you feel you're depressed or having diffi-culty coping. In the meantime, instead of eating when you're feeling out of sorts, be productive and try to stay on track with Urban Skinny.

If you're:

Lonely   Call a friend, make a lunch date, e-mail someone, join a running club or a book club.

Tired   Take a nap, walk around the block, take an exercise class, drink water, grab a coffee—not a candy bar. Food won't give you the energy you're craving. Sleep depri-vation impedes weight loss, so try to get some sleep.

Bored   Get a manicure, go shopping, read a book, go to the movies, play an online game, clean the closet—just do something!

Sad   Do what makes you feel happy, journal to see why you're sad, take a long walk, if you have a hobby that makes you feel better, do it. Garden, bake (but give it away), paint, draw, think of things you liked when you were little, volunteer.

Broke   Rob a bank (kidding), figure out your finances on paper and get a budget together. If you live alone, get a roommate, limit your cleaning lady, take fewer trips to Starbucks, log your expenses like you log your food, take subways not cabs, carpool, and decrease ordering in. If possible, get a part-time job at a place you love, like the gym or the wine store, and get fewer haircuts and pedicures. If you have to give up your trainer or pilates, give up the one that burns fewer calories.

Grieving   Nothing you eat will fill the void of grief. When you're grieving, you need to let yourself feel what you're feeling, so food doesn't become your coping mechanism. Grief is a big one, a true stressor—maybe give yourself a break and shift to weight maintenance and not weight loss until you cope with your loss. Do something in your loved one's honor, like plant a tree, but let yourself grieve.

Boy issues   If you get dumped, nothing is better revenge than looking fantastic. He's not sitting around moping, and neither should you. Stay on track, get dolled up, and get out there and be social. Eating more won't make him call.

Do what you have to do to feel empowered. If you're empowered, your chances of weight-loss success are greater. Nothing makes you kick ass more than feeling good, and twenty seconds working down the cheese platter won't empower you. When you're empowered, you're strong, and when you're strong, you have a good mindset. A positive mindset is a great weight-loss tool.

Urban Recap

Don't let the little things get to you and derail your weight-loss efforts. If you have emotional issues you can't get over, you can always get some professional help. When you see signs and are aware of them, use coping methods other than food to feel better.

Up Next

Setting weight-loss goals for yourself. It's not just about the scale. There are other ways to assess that shouldn't be ignored.

CHAPTER 11

It's Not All about
the Scale—
Setting Goals, Reaching Goals

Jack, network TV star, 6'3", 190 pounds, 11% body fat, super hot

Urban Challenge
Jack was leaner and fitter than most, but by model/actor standards, not enough. He needed to be ultra-ripped for some upcoming shirtless scenes.

Urban Surprise
Jack was a gym rat—He was working out hard every day for at least two hours, but he still couldn't pump out the six-pack he needed. He thought losing weight was the answer and set himself a goal of weighing 170 pounds.

Urban Insight
Muscle is denser than fat, so Jack had to learn to overlook the scale to a certain degree, and focus on the measure of body fat.

Jack always skipped breakfast, which was easily remedied, and he made sure he fueled his body with meals that included protein and fat every three or four hours. He upped his food intake instead of cutting it, eating 2000–2200 calories a day and always having a pre-workout meal. In just seven months, Jack was ripped; he had just 4% body fat, and—the big surprise for him—he weighed 180 pounds. Technically, Jack had dropped almost 14 pounds of fat, but since he gained almost 4 pounds of muscle, the net loss on the scale was 10 pounds.

Set Reasonable Goals and Be Patient

We spend our lives making goals, striving to achieve them, and either rejoicing when we accomplish them or feeling frustrated when we don't. If you want to be CEO by age thirty-five, or married by age thirty-two, or worth $500,000 by age twenty-nine, then you have something very specific to work towards. Weight-loss goals can't be that specific, but they can definitely exist. Take baby steps, don't feel defeated if you don't get there quickly, and have a solid understanding of the limits of your body before you set a goal for yourself. The key is to be happy with the small achievements along the way.

Don't Just Rely on the Scale

What should I weigh? That's a very tricky question. Your progress should be measured not only by what the scale says but also by your body-fat composition and your circumference measurements. You know not to put all your eggs in one basket, so don't put all your weight goals on the scale. The scale should not be the final word on your progress, because the scale weighs all of you—including muscle, bone, water, organs, and fat. It only tells you what your total weight is; it cannot differentiate muscle weight from fat or water weight. It is possible to lose weight and gain muscle and the scale won't budge. You may think you're not getting any leaner, but in fact you are. Your body will look smaller and feel thinner.

Body-Fat Assessment

Body-fat assessment will tell you if you are building muscle and losing fat (a good thing!). If you are a member of a gym, you can have a personal trainer check your body fat with skin calipers and get an idea of how much "fat" you actually have. If you don't have access to calipers, simply do your own measurements with a tape measure. Measure your hips, waist, bust, thighs, and arms before you start your weight-loss quest. After following Urban Skinny, measure again every month or so. If your measurements are smaller, then you are leaner—regardless of what the scale says.

A quick weight-goal guideline for women: 100 pounds for the first 5 feet of height and 5 pounds for every inch thereafter. For example: If you are 5'4" you should weigh 120 pounds: 100 pounds plus 20 pounds (4 inches x 5 pounds). But that is just a midpoint to work from. The range for any height is +/-10 percent, so the range for 5'4" can be 108–132 pounds. If you exercise you may be more muscular, or if you have a large frame shoot for the high end of the range—and vice versa if you have a small frame.

Reach to the Back of Your Closet

If your clothes are looser, you're smaller—scale or no scale. There is nobody sitting in your closet stretching your clothing. Pull something out of the back of the closet—like those skinny jeans you haven't been able to button up for a long time. If they fit, you're smaller, which is the goal. Don't worry about weight if you're getting to your goal of fitting into certain clothing. Muscle is denser than fat, which is why you may hear how much someone weighs and think, "Wow—she wears it well." You can be muscular (and weigh more) but still look like you've lost weight.

URBAN INSIGHT: If all of a sudden people are telling you that you look great, then you look great. It's working—you're getting leaner. Soak it in, use the praise as motivation to keep going, and enjoy how hot you look.

How Often Should I Weigh Myself?

For some people, the scale is as dreaded as the dentist. It's a temperamental gadget that can go up and down for no reason. Fluctuating after every sushi, Indian, Thai, or Mexican dinner, every airplane trip, and every hormonal cycle—it can make a girl crazy. Weighing in one to two times a week is plenty while you're losing weight. For the most accurate reading, weigh in first thing in the morning, naked, before you eat anything. If you weigh in at the gym or elsewhere, just be consistent about trying to weigh in at the same time of day on the same scale in order to accurately assess your progress.

Remember, if you had a salty dinner, are ovulating or mid-cycle, just got off a flight, haven't had a poop in days, had a bowl of pasta for dinner, or simply just ate a lot of food, then you may not like what you see on the scale the next morning. Your weight can fluctuate as much as five pounds for no real reason. It is very possible to see a five-pound increase on the scale the morning after a Mexican fiesta, but don't freak out! Give it a few days, go to the bathroom, drink lots of water, and weigh in again. You can't lose weight overnight, and it's certainly physically impossible to gain five pounds of fat while you slept for eight hours. Note: It's more normal to fluctuate than to not. If your scale reads the same daily despite a salty dinner of miso soup and sushi with soy sauce, then you may need to get a new scale.

How Quickly Should I Lose Weight?

The recommended weight-loss guidelines are set at a half to two pounds per week. If you are losing weight at a rate of more than two pounds in a week, you are not losing fat. You are losing muscle mass, glycogen (stored carbohydrates), and water. You don't want to lose lean muscle, since it is metabolically active tissue; you will wind up slowing down your metabolism, making it that much more challenging to keep losing weight. If you have a lot to lose, just shoot to drop 10 percent of your weight over the course of six months. You want to lose fat (you know, the dimples on your thighs).

What Should My Goal Weight Be?

A goal doesn't have to be scale or body-mass related. Maybe you want to be a size 6 or you want to fit into your fave old jeans from college.

Maybe you just want to weigh what you weighed on your wedding day. Pick anything that's important to you and go for it.

How Do I Know When It's Time to Stop Losing Weight?

Use a combination of things to kick into maintenance and stop losing: Use the weight chart for a goal weight, get into your BMI range (see charts below), like how you look, and feel good about the number on the scale. You can even use your skinny jeans—if you can zip them up, you have arrived.

Weight Chart

Height	Weight Range
5'0"	95–128
5'1"	98–132
5'2"	101–136
5'3"	104–140
5'4"	108–145
5'5"	111–150
5'6"	115–154
5'7"	118–159
5'8"	122–164
5'9"	125–169
5'10"	129–174
5'11"	133–179
6'0"	136–184
6'1"	140–189
6'2"	144–194
6'3"	148–199

Healthy Weight Ranges: Women stay at the lower end of the range and men at the higher end. Again, bone structure, muscle mass, and age should all be considered when checking your weight range.

BMI Chart

BMI Height (inches)	Normal						Overweight					Obese					
	19	20	21	22	23	24	25	26	27	28	29	30	31	32	33	34	35
									Body Weight (pounds)								
58	91	98	100	105	110	115	119	124	129	134	138	143	148	153	158	162	167
59	94	99	104	109	114	119	124	128	133	138	143	148	153	158	163	168	173
60	97	102	107	112	118	123	128	133	138	143	148	153	158	163	168	174	179
61	100	106	111	116	122	127	132	137	143	148	153	158	164	169	174	180	185
62	104	109	115	120	126	131	136	142	147	153	158	164	169	175	180	186	191
63	107	113	118	124	130	135	141	146	152	158	163	169	175	180	186	191	197
64	110	116	122	128	134	140	145	151	157	163	169	174	180	186	192	197	204
65	114	120	126	132	138	144	150	156	162	168	174	180	186	192	198	204	210
66	118	124	130	136	142	148	155	161	167	173	179	186	192	198	204	210	216
67	121	127	134	140	146	153	159	166	172	178	185	191	198	204	211	217	223
68	128	131	138	144	151	158	164	171	177	184	190	197	203	210	216	223	230
69	128	135	142	149	155	162	169	176	182	189	196	203	209	216	223	230	236
70	132	139	146	153	160	167	174	181	188	195	202	209	216	222	229	236	243
71	136	143	150	157	165	172	179	186	193	200	208	215	222	229	236	243	250
72	140	147	154	162	169	177	184	191	199	206	213	221	228	235	242	250	258
73	144	151	159	166	174	182	189	197	204	212	219	227	235	242	250	257	265
74	148	155	163	171	179	186	194	202	210	218	225	233	241	249	256	264	272
75	152	160	168	176	184	192	200	208	216	224	232	240	248	256	264	272	279
76	156	164	172	180	189	197	205	213	221	230	238	246	254	263	271	279	287

24.9—Watch out—you're getting to the high end of normal; start watching your intake.

28.5—Stop what you're doing and get back on track to lose some weight. You are carrying too much weight for your height right now.

30—Danger—be afraid; you are entering the Obese range and need to take steps to lose weight now.

Healthy weight ranges based on BMI: Normal: 18.5—24.9; Overweight: 25—29.9; Obese: 30—34.9; Morbidly obese: 35—39.9

Understanding the BMI Barometer

Normal

☐ Within a healthy weight range—good for you!

☐ Maybe you just want a ten-pound tweak.

☐ You're at minimal risk of developing heart disease, but if you're at the higher end of normal, you have a higher risk of developing diabetes.

☐ Women, if you're in this range but your waist measures more than thirty-five inches, you still need to lose weight.

☐ If you're at the high end of normal, stop further weight gain or lose a little.

> You can calculate your own BMI. Here's how:
> Divide weight in pounds by height in inches squared. Multiply by 703. BMI: wt (lbs) / ht^2 (inches) x 703

Overweight

☐ You might be in this range but have a muscular build, so don't panic; you may not be overweight.

☐ The first goal to set if you're sitting here is just to cross into the "normal" range.

☐ This is the point at which you start to increase your risk of cardiovascular disease and diabetes, as well as sleep apnea and other chronic diseases.

Obese

☐ Before you start any diet or exercise program, talk to your doctor.

☐ Make your first goal to get out of the obese category—take baby steps.

URBAN INSIGHT: You lose muscle when you age, which slows your metabolism. You can beat the clock, but you have to work harder as you get older. If you worked out three times a week to stay fit when you were twenty, you'll have to work out five times a week for the same results when you're forty.

BMI is not applicable to very muscular or fit individuals, since it may put them in the overweight range based on height and weight despite the fact that their body fat is very low. It is also not applicable for people who are very small framed with little muscle mass.

Even if your weight falls within the normal weight range, if your waist measurement exceeds thirty-five inches for women or forty inches for men, you still need to lose weight. Abdominal fat is an independent risk factor for developing cardiovascular disease and diabetes.

Urban Recap

Assess reaching your goals not just by watching the scale creep lower, but by measuring yourself, checking your BMI, fitting into your clothes, and having other people notice that you look fantastic. Set goals by picking clothing you want to wear again, a size you'd like to fit into, a weight-chart goal, a lower BMI, or just sculpted abs.

Up Next

If you haven't lost by now, and you're following the Urban Skinny plan, either something's physically wrong or you're doing something wrong. It's time to reassess, micro-focus, and figure out the problem.

CHAPTER 12

If All Else Fails,
Time to Reassess

Maggie, 33 years old, publicist

Urban Challenge
Maggie moved to the United States from Europe and, after being here for just a short while, gained weight. She wasn't used to the big portions restaurants here serve and she found herself eating out so much more than she ever did in Europe.

Urban Surprise
Maggie did well when she first started Urban Skinny. Very well, in fact. She got into a great routine, both with eating and working out. She was losing, even through the holidays, but come January she got stuck and couldn't budge the scale. She said she was doing the same thing she'd done before the holidays, and she was ultrafrustrated.

Urban Insight
Maggie had been so successful that she didn't think she needed to keep a food log anymore. She figured she was eating the same things she'd always eaten since starting Urban Skinny. It wasn't until she started logging again that she realized she'd slowly snuck extra calories

in and that, in fact, she wasn't eating as little as she thought she was. Amazingly, but not surprisingly, within five days of logging again, she'd already lost a pound. She quickly figured out that for her the only way to be accurate was to log. She got diligent about it and the pounds fell off again.

Angie, 45 years old, corporate recruiter

Urban Challenge
Angie had thyroid cancer and had her thyroid removed years before. She was taking medicine to treat the problem and kept up a regular exercise regimen, but she wasn't able to lose weight. Angie wanted to lose 15 pounds. She started Urban Skinny and dropped 11 pounds in four months. Then all of a sudden, without changing her habits, she packed it all back on and 20 more in a very short amount of time. She was 35 pounds from her goal and couldn't stop the weight gain.

Urban Surprise
Angie was no couch potato; she was training hard-core for Olympic-level triathlons. She worked out hard five times a week, logged her food intake, and was eating the right number of calories.

Urban Insight
Angie had been complaining of dry skin and constipation and that she was always tired and cold. Her periods were irregular. The endocrinologist changed up Angie's thyroid medication. She had a brief and slight dip in weight, and then out of nowhere it shot up even higher than it had been. She went back to the doctor, who told Angie she was insulin resistant and had to take additional medication for that. She was also put on a birth-control pill. She dumped 22 pounds of excess weight and is on track to reach her weight goal. She's under the doctor's supervision and takes her medicine regularly while continuing to train and eat properly.

Time for a Check-In

So you think you've done everything right, but you've arrived at this chapter still Urban, but not Urban Skinny. You got on the scale after week two and it hadn't moved. You ordered your dressing on the side and doubled up at the gym and still nothing. Don't be frustrated; just take a closer look at the situation. One of two things has happened:

1. What you're doing and what you think you're doing are not the same.
2. Something's wrong mentally or physically.

Most likely there's nothing wrong with you, so don't panic. More often, when people don't move the scale, they're not doing what they think they're doing. Let's go through this checklist first and make sure you're following Urban Skinny and are on target:

- ☐ **Are your portions off?** Unless you're measuring, you can't be sure. Weigh your protein and measure fats and starches whenever possible to make sure you're not overeating.
- ☐ **Is your math on track?** Are you adding everything up as you eat it, and logging it as you go along? Make sure you do. If you eat it, log it. That's the best way to be accurate. You can't go back and add it up at the end of the day— you'll forget the quick snack or the ingredients of your salad. It can't be said enough—if used correctly, the food log is your best weight-loss tool.
- ☐ **Could you be eating too many calories?** Go back and double-check what you're taking in and make sure it's no more than your allotted number. Check your activity level too, and be accurate when assessing it.
- ☐ **Are you really following the plan?** If you do something as small as not getting your dressing on the side, you could be adding 200 calories to your day without realizing it. Even

just 100 to 200 additional calories will keep you from losing weight. You won't gain, but you won't lose.

☐ **Are you eating breakfast?** There's no room for discussion here—eat it and get that metabolism moving. Don't save those calories for the end of the day.

☐ **Have you gotten a little too relaxed?** Maybe you had starch and wine at one sitting when you should have just chosen one or the other, or maybe you snuck a latte back in when you should have stuck to a cappuccino.

☐ **Are you drinking enough water?** If you're dehydrated you eat more, and if you're dehydrated your metabolism slows down over time. Your brain screws up signals between thirst and food . . . and likely you'll grab food in response.

Take the next seven to fourteen days and pretend you just learned Urban Skinny, so you're being ultracautious. Refocus your energy. Measure, hydrate, don't approximate. Write down every single thing that goes in your mouth right after you eat it. Humor us here—even a handful of M&M's. Also take your menstrual cycle into account, and watch your intake of salty foods. Don't be obsessive, just more meticulous and accurate. Tweak a little here and a little there—it might just be an extra 200 calories a day (a quick cookie you grabbed off someone's desk at work or a handful of almonds) that is adding up to prevent you from dropping the pounds. If you're being accurate, maybe you need to shave an extra 100 calories a day off of your intake for a week at a time to see if things start moving.

If you still don't lose and you're really being accurate and logging, take a mental checklist of your life. One of the following things could be causing your weight-loss block.

Stress

Okay, we're all stressed, we get it. We live in a big city and get tense when the train door shuts in our face or we are stuck in insane traffic.

Those are the little daily frustrations we all encounter but can't allow to hamper our weight loss. There are big-picture stresses, though, that could shut you down. There's stress and then there's stress. Real stress may mess with your levels of cortisol—a hormone that gets elevated when you're stressed. High levels of cortisol may cause weight gain, especially around your midsection. There's no magic pill for this; you just have to de-stress. Job loss, a death in the family, moving, divorce, or a break-up are major stress episodes. You could be eating right, exercising, and staying on track to a tee, but in these periods of truly serious stress the increased hormone levels may hinder you from losing weight. If you really can't focus on weight loss during a situation, that's okay—work on fixing the cause of your stress first. Be realistic and just aim to maintain your weight until you get through the crisis.

Sleep Deprivation

Whether you can't sleep because of the stress, or you're just not a good sleeper, for every hour less of sleep you get the greater your weight-loss challenge becomes. The guy who's getting seven hours of sleep will have an easier time than the gal who's only getting five. You need eight to nine hours a night. If you used to function on six and not have a weight issue, and all of a sudden you're only getting four, you'll be challenged. It's the decrease in sleep that's going to mess you up. When you're sleep deprived you're tired, and when you're tired you turn to food for energy. Think about how often you need an afternoon boost to get you through the day. Take a nap, not a sandwich. There's also an issue with two appetite hormones: leptin and grehlin. Grehlin is the hunger hormone and leptin is the hormone that signals satiety (feeling full and satisfied). When you don't get enough sleep, your grehlin levels increase, making you feel hungrier than usual. Leptin levels are lower than usual when you don't get enough sleep. Sleep deprivation is a three-fold disaster: You're left tired and looking for an energy boost, your hunger hormone is raging, and your "I'm full" hormone isn't working very well. If you can't take a nap, take a walk and get some fresh air instead of food, or at least be snack smart—make it a good choice like nuts and fruit.

Medical Issue

Medical issues that prevent weight loss—specifically an underactive thyroid—are more common in women than in men. Another problem some people develop is insulin resistance. Women may develop it because they have a condition called polycystic ovary syndrome. You can also develop insulin resistance if you've gained weight—especially in the midsection. Then it becomes a self-fulfilling prophecy: The weight gain triggers insulin resistance, which causes you to gain more weight. You need to lose weight to fix the insulin issue, but with the insulin issue it's almost impossible to lose weight. If you are insulin resistant, your doctor may prescribe medicine that will give you a fighting chance, but you'll have to use proper diet and exercise to beat it. One last thing to consider is that certain medications, like some antidepressants, beta-blockers for heart disease, steroids like prednisone, and certain anti-psychotics, will make weight loss difficult if not impossible. Consult a physician or endocrinologist if you're concerned one of these things is stopping your progress. If there's an underlying medical condition, you'll need to address it before trying to kick the pounds.

Urban Recap

Make sure you're following all of the Urban Skinny rules. Reassess. If you haven't lost weight, you may just need to refocus—you might simply need to reduce your calories. If you focus and you're not losing, keep in mind that stress or lack of sleep could be roadblocks. Finally, check with your doctor; something could be out of whack with your insulin levels or some medication you're on could be blocking your efforts.

Up Next

If you have been losing, and you've reached your goal, congratulations! But don't stop working. Maintaining is part of the challenge. You look fantastic, so let's keep it that way.

CHAPTER 13

You've Earned the
New Wallet, Not the Purse
(True Success Is
Keeping the Weight Off)

Elsa, 40 years old, weighed 171 pounds and had a BMI that bordered on obese.

Urban Challenge

Elsa made a boatload of cash on Wall Street and was able to "retire" before she reached the big 4-0. Elsa was a typical type-A worker. She juggled a high-powered job in finance that took her back and forth to Asia and kept her in the office twelve hours a day. She also battled a serious sweet tooth, especially a love of cookies and ice cream. While she doesn't go to an office on a regular basis now, she consults, sits on many boards of directors, and keeps a very busy social schedule.

Urban Surprise

Exercise was never Elsa's issue. Twice weekly she worked with a trainer, twice weekly she did cardio, and she walks two miles a day.

Urban Insight

Since Elsa retired at a young age, she was healthy and had time to really focus on her diet. She started keeping a food log and made sure that even though she cut her calories, her sweet cravings were still satisfied.

While on Urban Skinny she had a treat for her afternoon snack and was able to skip the late-night dessert binges. In less than six months, Elsa had gotten her BMI within the normal weight range and lost 37 pounds and 27 inches. A year after starting Urban Skinny, she had lost a total of 50 pounds. Over the next few years Elsa fluctuated, but only by 5 pounds. She never topped 127 pounds and never came close to the 171 pounds she'd weighed four years earlier. It was a challenge, but she kept her exercise routine up—hitting the gym for an hour at least five or six times a week. If her weight crept up, she started logging her food again. She also learned she couldn't eat the way she used to eat if the weight was going to stay off. These days, she makes her exercise more interesting by training for races, upping her speed, and beating her own personal records every time.

Keeping It Off

Congratulations, you've reached your weight goal! But don't go buy yourself a new Prada purse just yet, sister—you've only earned the wallet. You get the purse next year when you've kept all this weight off—that's when you've really earned it. Maintenance is the real Urban Challenge. Anybody can lose weight, but sadly almost everyone gains it back and then some. How many nights have you and your girlfriends lamented over margaritas the fact that you swore you'd never gain it back again, but you did? Trust us here—maintaining the weight loss, not just getting it off, is the finish line. You've worked so hard; don't trip up now.

> URBAN INSIGHT: When you lose weight, even if you do it the right way, you lose 75 percent fat mass and 25 percent muscle mass. Guess what: If you gain it back, you gain 100 percent back in fat. Meaning you might crawl back up to 150 pounds, but your 150-pound jeans don't fit because your body composition has changed.

It's likely most of the diet books and diets you've tried haven't taught you how to keep the weight off. In effect, they've dropped you at the curb without a map. But *Urban Skinny* isn't going to do that, because

Urban Skinny is as much a maintenance book as it is a weight-loss book. Leaving you without a maintenance plan would be like sending you down the red carpet without a stylist.

The steps are simple:

- ☐ **Stick to your calorie count.** Don't go back to eating how much you ate before you started Urban Skinny or you'll look like you used to look.

- ☐ **A diet low to moderate in fat will help you keep it off.** Fat should take up 25–30% of your daily calorie budget.

- ☐ **Keep logging your food.** You can take a more casual approach to it, but stay mindful of the calories you're taking in.

- ☐ **Don't shove your scale under the bed.** Keep stepping on it at least once a week so you know the score. Don't let your weight creep up.

- ☐ **Eat breakfast every single day without exception.**

- ☐ **Ease up on the computer and TV time.** If you're sitting on the couch, you're not on the treadmill.

- ☐ **Exercise is critical.** Don't cancel the gym membership.

Here's the skinny on working out: To prevent weight regain you have to stick to 60–90 minutes of moderate-intensity exercise—as in jogging or walking a fifteen-minute mile, swimming, biking, or yoga—most days of the week. If you jack up the intensity, you can decrease the duration and go for your massage a few minutes early. Turn that fifteen-minute walk into a ten-minute jog and make your leisurely bike ride a spin class. Exer-

You'll learn a lot about yourself as you aim to maintain. Everybody is wired differently. You may only need a few workouts a week, or only 30 minutes each time. You may need more. Keep your eye on the ball and make sure you monitor how your body adapts to exercise. Bottom line, you don't want the scale to go up, so do what you have to do. You're the best judge of how much exercise you'll need.

cise has to be your second job if you want to keep the weight off. You don't get paid cash, but the payoff is huge.

URBAN INSIGHT: If you walk up a flight of stairs with a knapsack on, your body is working harder than if you went up without the knapsack. The same concept applies to body fat. If you're smaller, you burn fewer calories because you're carrying less baggage. That means you've got to eat fewer calories to stay smaller. For every 20 pounds you lose, you need to shave about 150 calories from your daily intake.

Max Out Your Effort

You could maintain with diet alone if you keep those calories low. Or you could add more calories but go crazy at the gym burning them all off. Easier and proven to be successful: A healthy combo of both diet and exercise. You won't starve and you won't risk overuse injuries at the gym. Remember you may be able to maintain your weight loss if you just restrict your eating, but this is extremely difficult and has been proven to be not very successful long-term.

URBAN INSIGHT: When walking in New York City, twenty city blocks is a mile, which translates to 100 burned calories. Four crosstown blocks is a mile. Start walking. If you don't have blocks to measure, grab a cheap pedometer or order one on your iPhone. If you clock 2,000 steps, that's approximately a mile. You might find the pedometer keeps you motivated as you see how your walking adds up throughout the day.

Make Time for Exercise

Don't say you don't have time for working out—you have to make some time. Clock your 60–90 minutes all at once or in little bits. Jump off the subway a few stops early or park your car at the back of the lot so you do more walking. Get out of bed just ten minutes early and do some sit-ups and push-ups. But make time to move. Even CEOs who run multibillion-dollar conglomerates find time to hit the treadmill—even if it's at 5:00 a.m. Not a morning person? No excuse. DVR and TiVo can record your shows so you won't get behind on *Survivor,* so you can take a quick boxing class after work and watch later. Or in case you pretended not to notice, most treadmills at the gym have televisions.

Hard Numbers

So how much can you actually eat to maintain all the hard work you've just put in? Tweak here; it's not an exact science. Try this: Add 100 a day to the daily calorie allotment you used when losing weight. So if you ate 1500 calories a day to lose weight, eat 1600. Try this for a week and then weigh yourself.

After the first week, if you're still losing weight or haven't gained weight, add another 100 calories a day. By the third week, if you still haven't gained even one pound, add another 100 calories.

Keep adding 100 calories each week until you see the scale go up—then stop adding calories. Stay at that count for the next week or two and if your weight stabilizes, you've reached your maintenance intake amount. If your scale goes up more, go down another 100 calories.

Remember, some of you may only get another 200 calories a day and others will get 500. If it's difficult for you to live with that calorie amount, up your gym time and you may be able to add a few more calories.

URBAN INSIGHT: A lot of people think that when they reach their goal weight they get to take a break. They rework that extra cookie into their day and slowly all the good habits they've learned in order to lose the weight go out the window. People think weight loss was a project and an end has been reached. The truth is there is no end. You don't get a break. The science doesn't change just because that little black dress finally fits and you look like a siren at the party. The party is just beginning, but the calories don't all of a sudden stop counting because you look hot.

Healthy Eating

Just because a food is healthy doesn't mean it's low in calories. Until this point, we've been talking budget, balance, and portions. We really haven't been on you about the principles of good nutrition. You used plan B when you had to and grabbed a donut; you had 500 calories' worth of chocolate one night and called it dinner. You logged your food, you counted calories, you split the day's food up properly. On occasion, you may have had a relatively unhealthy day, but you stuck to your number. That's why you lost weight—it's been all about the calories. We wanted you to be able to live your life and still hit your weight goal. Job one was living within your calorie budget. That's been fine—you got the weight off—and on occasion you can still spend your calories in a wacky way as long as you don't do it every day.

But now you don't want to be that unhealthy skinny person, so only counting calories is no longer enough. We didn't let you do the cabbage diet, but we're not letting you do the donut diet either, even if you still only eat 1500 calories a day. It's time to make some long-term investments in what you put into your body that will pay back like dividends, but in ways that keep you lean and healthy.

URBAN INSIGHT: Don't celebrate reaching your weight goal with a fabulous dinner. Food is not a reward or a punishment. Buy some kick-ass boots instead. Or some new Nikes! Or a little black dress. Or a new pair of skinny jeans. . . .

Give the new you a fighting chance by making healthy choices. It's not just for your health; you can also stretch that calorie budget a lot further with good picks. You may have heard this all before, but try to work these basics into your day as you set off on your maintenance journey.

- ❒ **Fruits and veggies:** Make each meal colorful. Add red and yellow peppers to the salad, throw blueberries on your cereal, slice a nice tomato and slap it on your turkey sandwich—or skip the sandwich and have a salad for lunch. The deeper, the darker, the richer the color, the more nutrients. Eat 5–9 servings of fruits and vegetables a day. Think the size of a tennis ball or one cup when trying to figure out a serving of fruit, which is about 75–100 calories a hit. A cup of raw leafy greens or half a cup of cooked veggies makes a serving and calories are almost zippo. Heavy up on the veggies because you get more bang for your calorie buck.

> The darker, the richer, the deeper the color of your vegetables, the better— they pack more vitamins, minerals, and antioxidants. For example, spinach not only looks better than iceberg lettuce, it's also better for you.

☐ **Grains and starches:** Think whole grains. Half of the starches you eat in a day should fit this bill. (White flour is passé anyway.) Quinoa, sweet potatoes, and brown rice are also fashionable picks. A diet high in fiber may reduce your risk of certain diseases and cancer, and (the extra bonus for weight management) fiber is filling. Eat 25 to 30 grams of fiber a day. Read labels, because some whole-grain bread is made with enriched flour, which is processed and low in fiber.

☐ **Protein:** Keep it lean, just like your new body. Stick with chicken, fish, and lean cuts of beef and pork. Limit the filet mignon, ribs, and porterhouse. Beef products are not only higher in calories, but higher in saturated fat and cholesterol, too. Including protein keeps your appetite in check.

☐ **Fats:** Just like all those first dates, fats can be good, bad, and absolutely forgettable. Good fats are mono- and polyunsaturated (found in olive oil, avocado, nuts, salmon, flax seeds, and canola oil). Bad fats are in butter, bacon, whole milk, cheese, ice cream, beef, sausage, skin-on chicken, and coconut and palm kernel oils (found in banana chips and other yogurt-coated treats). Must-never-meet-again fats are trans fats (otherwise known as partially hydrogenated oils), which can be found in margarine, many brands of commercially prepared crackers, cookies, and baked goods, and fried fast food (except in cities in which they've been banned). Good or bad, all fats are high in calories, so eat in moderation.

☐ **Water:** Dehydration makes you eat more because your brain's signals get confused. Chronic dehydration decreases your energy level and slows your metabolism. Don't wait until you're thirsty; once you're thirsty, you're already dehydrated.

Urban Recap

Maintenance is a lifelong project. Keep exercising, logging, and stepping on the scale. Tweak your calories so you know if you can eat a few more after you've lost, but if your weight creeps up, you're eating too many calories. If you eat like you used to, you'll look like you used to. Shift to a healthy eating plan. You may have been winging it to get the weight off, but to maintain and be healthy eat high fiber, whole grains, lean proteins, and fruits and veggies.

Up Next

A fabulous, healthy, hot new you!

Glossary

Amino Acids

Amino acids are the building blocks of protein. There are 20 amino acids needed to construct protein molecules, some of which the body can manufacture and others that must be obtained from the foods in one's diet. Another good reason to include a little protein in each meal.

Body Mass Index (BMI)

A way to gauge your body weight in relation to your height. BMI is used as a screening tool to identify possible weight problems and is used to determine the federal government's official definitions of adult overweight and obesity. For most people, a BMI between 18.5 and 24.9 indicates a healthy weight. A BMI of 25 or above is considered overweight. Obesity is defined as a BMI of 30 or above. The BMI is a general guide and may be inappropriate for some very muscular people or those with very little muscle mass.

Calories

Like you haven't heard this term before . . . We watch and count them all day long. A calorie is a measure of the energy of food. For example, a medium apple contains approximately 100 calories. A calorie is also a measure of energy expenditure. For example, walking a mile on the treadmill burns, on average, 100 calories. Weight management is based on the simple equation of calories in versus calories out.

Dietary Fat

One of the three classes of macronutrients that make up our diet. Fat has many roles in the body, including being a great source of energy, providing essential fatty acids such as omega-3 polyunsaturated fat and omega-6 polyunsaturated fat, and serving as a carrier for the absorption of the fat-soluble vitamins A, D, E, and K. Total fat intake should be between 20 and 35 percent of total calories. Polyunsaturated and monounsaturated fats should be the primary sources of dietary fat.

Dietary Fiber

Found only in plant foods like whole grains, fruits, nuts, and vegetables, fiber consists of certain carbohydrates our bodies cannot digest or absorb. Unlike other carbohydrates, fiber is eliminated from the body, taking with it waste products the body doesn't need. There are two types of fiber, soluble and insoluble. The recommended daily intake of fiber is 25–35 grams.

Soluble Fiber

Soluble fiber is found mostly in beans, oats, barley, and psyllium seed. It can help to lower cholesterol levels and control insulin levels, thereby reducing risk for the development of cardiovascular disease and diabetes in some people.

Insoluble Fiber

Insoluble fiber is found mostly in whole-grain breads and cereals, including wheat and corn bran. Insoluble fiber is known as "roughage," which keeps things moving along the digestive tract.

Monounsaturated Fatty Acid

An unsaturated fat found primarily in plant foods, including olives and olive oil, canola oil, and peanuts and peanut oil. These fats are liquid at room temperature. A diet rich in monounsaturated fats has been shown to decrease risk of cardiovascular disease because of the cholesterol-lowering effect.

Net-Impact Carbohydrates

Food companies created the term "net-impact carbohydrates" to give their products more shelf appeal. Net-impact carbs result from replacing wheat flour with soy flour or adding fiber, sugar alcohols, or fat. According to experts, these compounds don't increase blood sugar the way other carbohydrates do.

Polyunsaturated Fatty Acid

This unsaturated fat is found in the greatest amount in plant foods such as soybeans, safflower, corn, and sunflower oils. Heart-healthy omega-3 fatty acids, which are found in tuna, salmon, sardines, herring, and flax seeds, are also a source of polyunsaturated fatty acids. These fats are liquid at room temperature. A diet rich in polyunsaturated fats has been shown to decrease risk of cardiovascular disease because of the cholesterol-lowering effect.

Protein

One of the three classes of macronutrients that make up our diet. Protein is the major structural component of all cells in the body, essentially our body's "building blocks." A common misconception is that just by eating protein you can increase your muscle mass. That is only half true. Although protein is necessary to build muscle tissue, muscle mass cannot be increased without a regular exercise routine. Dietary protein sources include fish, chicken, beef, eggs, beans, cheese, and nuts.

Saturated Fatty Acid

This type of fat is found in the greatest amounts in foods from animals, such as fatty cuts of meat, poultry with the skin, whole-milk products, and lard. These fats are also found in two plant sources: palm kernel and coconut oils. These fats are solid at room temperature, just like they would be "solid" in your arteries. As a result, they can raise total cholesterol levels and in particular LDL (bad) levels, therefore increasing risk of cardiovascular disease. Saturated fat should account for 7–10 percent of total calories.

Trans Fatty Acid

A fatty acid that has been produced by a process called hydrogenation, which converts a liquid oil to a more solid oil, thereby making it more stable. Trans fats are naturally present in meat and dairy products; however, the main sources of trans fats in the United States are partially hydrogenated (hardened) oils found in foods such as cookies, crackers, pastries, and fried foods. The government and food industry are working together to reduce or eliminate trans fats in foods, since they wreak such havoc on our cholesterol levels. Trans fats not only raise levels of LDL (the bad cholesterol) but also decrease HDL (the good cholesterol), thereby increasing our risk of heart disease with a double punch.

References, Resources, and Tools

American Dietetic Association (ADA)
120 South Riverside Plaza, Suite 2000
Chicago, IL 60606-6995
800-877-1600
www.eatright.org

American Heart Association (AHA)
National Center
7272 Greenville Avenue
Dallas, TX 75231
800-242-8721
www.americanheart.org

Centers for Disease Control and Prevention (CDC)
1600 Clifton Road
Atlanta, GA 30333
800-CDC-INFO (232-4636)
www.cdc.gov

National Institutes of Health (NIH)
9000 Rockville Pike
Bethesda, MD 20892
301-496-4000
www.nih.gov

The National Weight Control Registry (NWCR)
Brown Medical School/Miriam Hospital
Weight Control and Diabetes Research Center
196 Richmond Street
Providence, RI 02903
800-606-NWCR (6927)
www.nwcr.ws

U.S. Department of Health and Human Services
200 Independence Avenue SW
Washington, DC 20201
877-696-6775
www.hhs.gov

Urban Skinny
www.urbanskinny.com

Weight Management
A Dietetic Practice Group
American Dietetic Association
www.wmdpg.org

Acknowledgments

A huge thanks goes to an early believer—our agent, Maura Teitelbaum at Abrams Artists Agency. Thanks for providing us with some seriously no-nonsense advice and advancing our project faster than we could say "Urban Skinny." Much gratitude goes to our fabulous editor at GPP, Lara Asher, for her tremendous encouragement, genius edits, and all the "I love this section!" notes. You made the process such a pleasure, and we're thrilled that you embraced and loved our concept as much as we did. Thanks to our crack legal team, Ann Marie Croswell, Elizabeth Corradino, and David McGrail, whose contributions were critical. To Jacqueline Krikorian (Stephanie's sister) for her comprehensive copy-edits: Your time was much appreciated. That little tip about backing up our work was also a good one. Thanks for facilitating and thanks for always being the biggest cheerleader (not just for this book). To Amy Fond, who can eat anything she wants, but still took the time to painstakingly read drafts of *Urban Skinny* and make great suggestions, and who now orders her dressing on the side. And thanks to Janet Lee-Jackson for your eleventh-hour copy-edits during that rainy weekend in Montauk. We'd also like to thank Reebok Sports Club/NY, Maureen Rooney and her team, Pamela Harris, Amy Wigler, Elizabeth Chandler, Kate Navin, Gwyn Osnos, Sarah Powers, Karen Merz, Steve Frank, and Gary Parr for early guidance, referrals, and suggestions, and Lori Berkowitz for her tremendous photography skills. Amber Milt, Jessica Shapiro, and Janine Spaulding—thanks for the early reads.

Special thanks from Danielle:
To my husband, Michael: Thanks for your patience and being cool with my time away. Your understanding, insight, support, and encouragement mean the world to me. Thanks for knowing when I really needed a compliment and for learning to sweetly phrase your constructive criticism. I love you *this* much. To my parents, my sisters, Lisa and Heather, and my brother, Ricky—you guys are the best. To my nieces Sydney and Ciara—I love you, and make sure you eat your veggies. I couldn't have

done this without my mom, Linda Schupp, always telling me I could do anything and for giving me a lifetime of unconditional love. I'd especially like to thank all of my clients. You've all given me the opportunity to peer into your different lives. You've trusted me with your stresses and lifes' challenges and let me live your many crazy experiences along with you, through your food logs and our chats. Without all of you exciting and interesting people, there would be no Urban Skinny to write about.

Special thanks from Stephanie:
To my mom and dad, Julie and Don Krikorian, who are unquestionably the most amazing parents in the world. I thank you from the bottom of my heart for your endless love, encouragement, and emotional and financial support, and for always saying, "Give it a shot—what have you got to lose?" To my sister, Jennifer, for decades of laughs (think "menu on fire"), and to my niece and home-girl Katie—you are the biggest joy in all of our lives. Thanks for sending me a notebook in which to write my book. Much gratitude to my dear friend Erin Turner for leaving me a trail of bread crumbs to follow and to Karyn Ohlson and Gina Saudin for years of support on everything, but especially this book. And lots of love to all of my wonderful friends for asking, analyzing, listening, questioning, contributing, and encouraging. I'm exceedingly lucky to have you all in my life. Thanks for letting every dinner out over the past two years be an Urban Skinny food analysis.

Index

About the Authors

Danielle Schupp has been a registered dietitian and a sports nutritionist at Reebok Sports Club/NY, one of Manhattan's hottest gyms, for 12 years. Danielle has appeared in *Shape, Forbes, Marie Claire, Redbook,* and *US Weekly.* She's been on *Live! with Regis and Kelly* and several local New York stations. She loves to travel, collect antiques, and—much to her husband's chagrin—buy really expensive decorative pillows. Pilates is her favorite weekend workout. Danielle earned her degree in nutritional science/dietetics from Cornell University and completed her dietetic internship at Columbia University. She is accredited by the American Dietetic Association and holds a Weight Management certification. She lives in Manhattan with her candy-loving husband, Michael.

Stephanie Krikorian is a globetrotting TV journalist and writer who has traveled to six continents. She's done stories on everything from the unrest in Israel to the Grammy Awards' red carpet. She's a travel junkie, foodie, wine enthusiast, and yoga nut. Once a week, she takes a pole-dancing class. She's amused by the fact that her first book is about weight loss considering how hard she battles the genes she was born with so she can fit into the jeans she bought last week. Stephanie studied English and drama at the University of Western Ontario and holds a Master of Science in TV, radio, and film from Syracuse University. She was born and raised in Canada, where her family still lives. She currently resides in Manhattan and loves it.